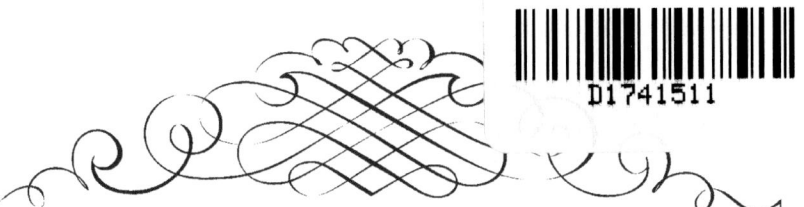
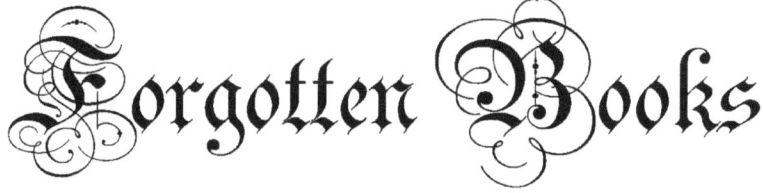
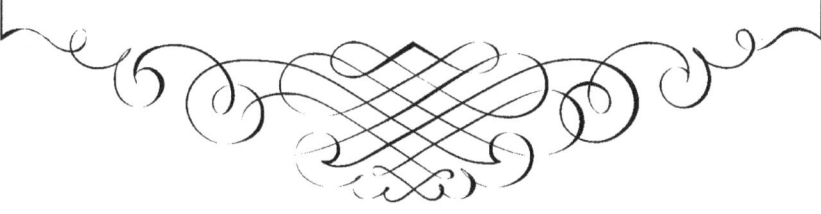

ISBN 978-1-5278-7685-9
PIBN 10906286

1 MONTH OF
FREE
READING

at
www.ForgottenBooks.com

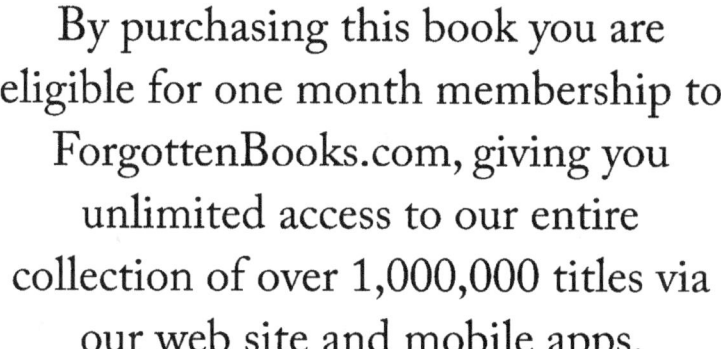

By purchasing this book you are eligible for one month membership to ForgottenBooks.com, giving you unlimited access to our entire collection of over 1,000,000 titles via our web site and mobile apps.

To claim your free month visit:

www.forgottenbooks.com/free906286

English
Français
Deutsche
Italiano
Español
Português

www.forgottenbooks.com

Mythology Photography **Fiction**
Fishing Christianity **Art** Cooking
Essays Buddhism Freemasonry
Medicine **Biology** Music **Ancient
Egypt** Evolution Carpentry Physics
Dance Geology **Mathematics** Fitness
Shakespeare **Folklore** Yoga Marketing
Confidence Immortality Biographies
Poetry **Psychology** Witchcraft
Electronics Chemistry History **Law**
Accounting **Philosophy** Anthropology
Alchemy Drama Quantum Mechanics
Atheism Sexual Health **Ancient History**
Entrepreneurship Languages Sport
Paleontology Needlework Islam
Metaphysics Investment Archaeology
Parenting Statistics Criminology
Motivational

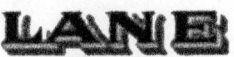
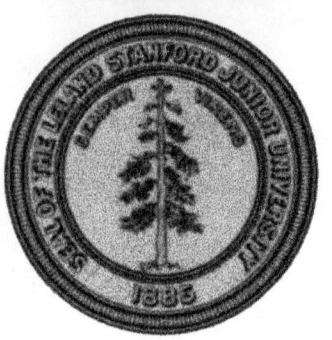

Dr A Jacobi
with the kind regards of
L. Duncan Bulkley

n 24. 1906

THE INFLUENCE OF THE MENSTRUAL FUNCTION ON CERTAIN DISEASES OF THE SKIN.

THE

Influence of the Menstrual Function on Certain Diseases of the Skin

BY

L. DUNCAN BULKLEY, A.M., M.D.

Physician to the New York Skin and Cancer Hospital,
Consulting Physician to the New York Hospital, Consulting Dermatologist
to the Randall's Island Hospitals, to the Manhattan Eye and Ear
Hospital, and to the Hospital for Ruptured and Crippled, etc.

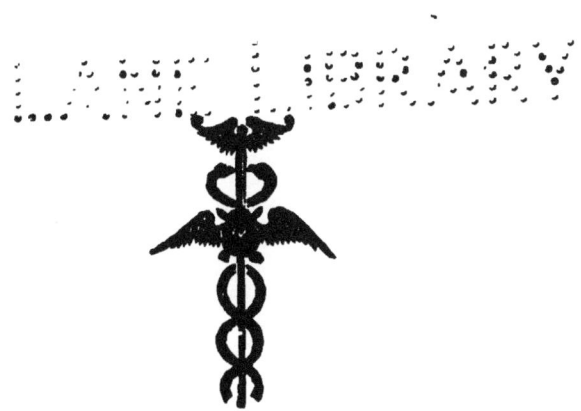

NEW YORK
REBMAN COMPANY
1123 BROADWAY

1906

LONDON
REBMAN LIMITED
129 SHAFTESBURY AVENUE

LAME LIBRARY

Printed in America

PREFACE.

For very many years medical thought has been busy seeking for the ultimate cause of disease, and various theories have arisen to account for the occasional relationships which have been observed between disease or disorder of different organs composing the human frame. Scattered references have been made, from time to time, in regard to the apparent influence of sexual disturbances in inducing pathological conditions in various parts of the body, but thus far no very full study of many of them has been made.

Repeated observations, however, occur in books and articles on diseases of the skin, and elsewhere, as to the apparent influence of uterine and ovarian disease in certain cutaneous disorders, many of which are very striking and conclusive; and all who see much of practice must at times have noticed such occurrences; but as yet relatively few definite and positive facts have been ascertained and recorded in regard to the relation of menstruation as a process as affecting the system, and no wholly satisfactory explanation of the effects occasionally seen in the skin has been presented.

My attention was first directed to the subject many years ago by the interesting brochure of Danlos, "Etude sur La Menstruation, au point de vue de son influence sur les Maladies Cutanées," Paris, 1874, and I at once verified many of his observations. Nearly twelve years ago I began a small note book, in which I have occasionally recorded instances where a relationship between the menstrual function and various diseases of the skin was particularly evident, and have been struck by the frequency with which this occurred, when investigation was instituted in regard to the mode of performance of this function. The connection was especially noticed in regard to acne, and so frequently did this occur that I ceased to make particular record of these cases: the same is partially true in regard to eczema. But as years went on I observed now and again many instances where various eruptions were markedly influenced in this manner, until, at the time of writing, the recorded observations amount to ninety-one, with fresh and often very striking instances continually presenting themselves; this does not include very many cases of acne and eczema, not specially recorded, where the influence of menstruation was observed to a lesser or greater degree.

The subject was presented briefly five years ago, (Trans. Medical Society State of New York, 1901), and since that time over half the cases have been observed and material from literature largely collected.

In attempting to analyze the material at hand, I am conscious that the difficult task has been but imperfectly done. Much more careful observation is necessary, as well as clinical and laboratory research, before the subjects and theories presented can be accepted as fully decided. But the present study may, perhaps, serve as a stimulus to others, and as a basis upon which abler hands may build more certain and definite material, until we know more perfectly the true nature of the mysterious "menstrual cycle," and its effects upon the various portions of the body, including the skin.

531 Madison Avenue, New York.

CONTENTS.

CHAPTER I.

GENERAL CONSIDERATIONS.

CHAPTER II.

CLINICAL RECORDS.

CHAPTER III.

ANALYSIS OF FACTS AND THEORIES.

CHAPTER IV.

TREATMENT.

THE INFLUENCE OF THE MENSTRUAL FUNCTION ON CERTAIN DISEASES OF THE SKIN.

CHAPTER I.

GENERAL CONSIDERATIONS.

The natural life of the human female presents three stages: 1. That from birth to puberty; 2. The period of menstruation and possible child bearing; and 3. That of the menopause. Each of these stages has relations to disorder and disease of various organs, which may differ greatly in different individuals, as is abundantly shown by clinical experience.

The study of sexual influences in many directions is a most interesting and instructive one, which has been far too little pursued, although success in practice may very often depend largely upon the right recognition of the relations involved.

It is the purpose of the present study to consider one single aspect of the subject, during the child-bearing period, namely, that relating to the menstrual function; and again it is limited to only a very small section of this, to wit, its relation at times to certain diseases of the skin. The menstrual function is here understood to represent the normal exhibition of that certain mysterious peculiarity of the female life, whose ultimate end is the reproduction of the species. We shall not attempt to consider the effect of derangement or disease of the sexual organs on the skin.

It would be quite out of place to attempt to enter here at all fully into the nature or cause of the menstrual flow, or its relation to ovulation, about which authorities are still divided. We may, however, accept the view which has been fairly proven by Putnam Jacobi, Stevenson, and Reinl, and summarized by Hirst,[61] that "a woman in her full sexual vigor seems to pass through a series of cyclical changes, of each of which the menstrual period is the climax." Or, as another writer[67] puts it, "menstruation is not a local process, but a general physiological action, a menstrual cycle finding its local expression in the generative organs."

Putnam Jacobi[68] has shown that the urea is generally increased in the urine before the appearance of the menses, and falls during and after; that the temperature is raised about one degree; that the pulse is accelerated, and that the sphygmograph shows increased arterial tension during the seven to nine days preceding menstruation, and reaches a minimum point in from one to four days after its cessation.

Weir Mitchell[85] has found that "in many women who are not perfectly well, there is a notable loss of weight at every menstrual period, and marked gain between these times," an observation which was made many years before by Sanctorius.[103]

This latter observation has recently been very strikingly verified by Belfield[6] from a study of four healthy, unmarried women. He found a progressive increase of the weight, from 2½ to 5 pounds, during several days, especially the first, preceding the menstrual flow. The climax of this gain is immediately followed by the rapid loss of a large part, perhaps one-half (often within 8 to 16 hours) and then a more gradual loss of the remainder, extending over several days, the menstrual flow beginning during the rapid loss of weight. He regards the pre-menstrual gain as due, not to increased ingestion of food, but to diminished excretion, especially of water. The rapid loss of weight is due, not to abstinence from food, (nor, of course, to the trifling loss of menstrual blood), but to rapid excretion, notably of carbon dioxid and water. For two days preceding the climax in weight there is often marked torpidity of the bowels and scantiness of the urine; while, with the decline in weight, excretion by the bowels and kidneys, as well as by skin and lungs, is notably increased. He has also noted a rise in temperature of about 1° F. during the increase in weight and a sudden fall after the crest of the weight wave is passed.

The well-recognized changes in the thyroid gland during menstruation also point to the cyclic condition of the system which is under consideration. Whether a hyper-secretion of the thyroid, which has been stated to take place normally at each menstrual epoch, is a contributing element to the "cyclic change" or is a result of it, cannot now be determined. The thyroid often enlarges during menstruation, and many of the unpleasant general symptoms which sometimes appear during this time are similar to those induced by excessive thyroid feeding, when given medically.

Ewing[41] gives the results of a number of observers who show that normal menstruation reduces the hemoglobin 4 to 15 per cent., and the red cells 220,543, while the leucocytes are slightly increased. "In the inter-menstrual period the red cells slowly increase, reaching a maximum three days before the succeeding flow."

Keiffer[68] quoting Charrin's demonstration that a woman's blood at the moment of the menses possesses its maximum of toxicity, believes that the various troubles recorded in different organs, in connection with menstruation, are traceable to an auto-intoxication of genital origin. In support of this he notices the fact that so many of these disturbances pass away when a more complete sexual life, as in matrimony, comes to develop, regulate and complete its functional activity.

The nervous system should also be taken very largely into account in considering the influence of menstruation on certain diseases of the skin; as would be expected in consideration of the enormous nervous supply of the sexual apparatus and its intimate relations with the sympathetic ganglia. But it is especially indicated by the marvellous neurotic phenomena affecting other organs, which have from time to time been reported in connection with disturbance of the sexual functions, often recurring with each menstrual epoch. Tilt[114] attributes the various phenomena attending change of life to ganglionic influence, and from the relations of the sympathetic nervous system to disease, as shown by Long Fox[42] it can be readily understood how the various phenomena may occur, through the abundant supply of ganglionie elements to the sexual system.

Engelmann[89] dwells strongly on the reflex character of certain phenomena which occur in the skin and other organs, in connection with menstruation and sexual disease, which he classes as hystero-neuroses. Later the attempt will be made to analyze the subject, in regard to the manner in which the various skin conditions to be mentioned are influenced by menstruation in each of these three directions.

There are, as is well known, two special periods at which functional disturbances in other organs are most prone to occur in connection with menstruation; namely, the period of development, or puberty, and that of cessation, or the menopause.

The changes in the mental and physical condition which attend the developing period of puberty are well known to all. The rounding out of the form, with increase of adipose tissue, the growth of hair on certain parts, and the readiness to flush or blush, and also to perspire, all indicate activity in the skin, which favors pathological changes.

The period of the menopause also presents special physiological and pathological conditions which have a natural bearing on certain diseases of the skin. As the "menstrual cycle" ceases to exist, slowly or rapidly, there may be many disturbances of various kinds in different organs, indicating the disturbance of the system from the arrest of this cyclical habit of body, indicated by menstruation. All are familiar with the flushes and perspirations so common at this time, which Tilt[114] found in over fifty per cent. of women.

We note also the tendency to growth of hair on the face, and to obesity.

But while disorders of some organs are, perhaps, more common at puberty and the menopause, it is a mistake to suppose that the periods of monthly menstruation between are without effect, at least as far as concerns the skin; for daily experience demonstrates that with each recurrent menstruation there may be, and very frequently is, a very perceptible, and sometimes a very considerable influence exerted on many skin lesions. This I have observed in hundreds of instances, both in those with and in those without appreciable uterine or ovarian disease.

CHAPTER II.

CLINICAL RECORDS.

The clinical aspect of the subject under consideration is a very large one, and it is difficult to do justice to the great amount of material, illustrating the relations under consideration, which is found in literature, as indicated in the appended bibliography. But while presenting personal experience the attempt will also be made to include such matter as will give as complete a consideration of the subject as possible.

In a book of special record, which I have kept for over ten years, I find memoranda relating to 91 patients in private practice in whom striking facts in regard to a connection between the menstrual function and various skin affections have appeared to be particularly worthy of note. In dozens of other cases, especially of acne and eczema, during past years, the same relations have been observed, but in the pressure of office work it is difficult to remember always to record scientific facts in a manner in which they can be utilized.

These ninety-one patients, of whom special note was made, suffered from twenty different diseased conditions of the skin; in many instances the cases were followed through a period of many months, or even years, and the influence of menstruation was observed again and again. In most instances the special record was made because the patient herself noticed or called attention to the menstrual influence manifested.

1. **Acne.** The eruption which most frequently and strongly demonstrates the influence of the menstrual function is acne, in its various forms. This is so well recognized by writers generally that it is not necessary to cite the many allusions to it, or quote the numerous illustrations which abound in literature.

Writers from the oldest times have mentioned the appearance of acne during the development of puberty, and many casually mention its recurrence or increase at each menstrual epoch. Hebra,[58] who is so often regarded as a localist, says "in certain persons acne rosacea exists only during the week preceding menstruation," also "the unquestioned increase and diminution of the phenomena of acne rosacea very frequently show its relations to the functions of the genital apparatus very clearly."

So commonly have I observed its occurrence that I have long since ceased to make any particular note of cases in the special record just referred to, but I find a number of striking instances there entered.

In many cases I find it recorded that the eruption was observed to be intensely aggravated just before the menstrual epoch, or at its beginning, and that it at once improved when the flow was well established. In a number of instances it was recorded that acne lesions appeared only just before or during menstruation, and repeatedly in asking patients in regard to its occurrence then, they have replied somewhat thus: "Of course, every woman knows that such an eruption is liable to appear then, and can often foretell the monthly sickness in this way."

In an analysis which I made some years ago[15] of fifteen hundred acne cases, it was found that 67.4 per cent., or over two-thirds of them occurred in females. In the notes of five-hundred-and-ten of these cases there were found references to the menstrual function, and in but one hundred and ninety-one cases was it recorded as perfectly normal. In regard, however, to the direct influence of the menstrual function on the skin, in no less than one hundred and fifty (150) instances it was recorded that the eruption was worse at or near the monthly period; in seventy-nine (79) cases it was aggravated *during* each menstrual epoch, and in five (5) of them it appeared only at this time; in fifty-two (52) cases it generally became worse *before* the appearance of the menses, and in fourteen (14) it was worse *after* the occurrence of the menstrual flow.

In some of the cases there was no marked uterine derangement, but very many patients exhibited various disturbances of the menstrual function, amenorrhœa, dysmenorrhœa, and menorrhagia; displacements, ulceration, endometritis, and pelvic cellulitis were occasionally recorded; ovarian congestion and neuralgia were frequently recognized; and leucorrhœa was noted as a common occurrence, together with the many aches and pains and distressing conditions recognized as associated with and more or less dependent upon deranged menstruation.

In many instances it was recorded that when the acne was found to be worse, or to have recurred, menstrual disturbance had also returned. In discussing my paper on acne before the New York Academy of Medicine in 1872, the late Dr. Peaslee remarked, that when he observed acne on the chin of females he almost always found some menstrual difficulty; this observation I have verified in scores of cases since that time. The connection between acne simplex and puberty, and acne rosacea and the menopause, is a matter of daily observation.

2. **Eczema.** The influence of the menstrual flow upon eczema is often exhibited in a very striking

manner, as has been confirmed by numerous observers. Danlos[27] has recorded some striking cases, where the eruption appeared with each menstrual epoch, either as an acute outbreak or as an exacerbation of a chronic state. Vrain[120] corroborates the same, especially dwelling on the concurrence of eczema with the first appearance of the menses and with pregnancy; and Goutry[48] reports a case of eczema in which at each menstrual epoch there were distinct exacerbations. Joseph[66] has reported an interesting case in a woman, aged thirty, who had eczema of the head, which while it disappeared almost entirely in the inter-menstrual period always returned at the menses. She had been married thirteen years, and had two children. Menstruation was always regular, every four weeks, and lasted four or five days, during the first three of which she lost a large amount of blood; she had chronic metritis and antiflexion.

Many writers note casually the influence of menstruation, or of uterine or ovarian disease on eczema, and Hebra[57] is very strong in his statements regarding the occurrence of eczema in connection with and depending upon menstrual disturbances and pregnancy, and at the menopause; he adds, "We simply record the fact, which is confirmed by many observations, and leave it to the future to demonstrate the closer relationship of these conditions." Rayer[97] says "amenorrhœa and dysmenorrhœa sometimes exercise a remarkable influence on the development of eczema."

The influence of the menstrual function in eczema is pretty clearly seen when an analysis of a considerable number of cases exhibiting this eruption is made. In a study of eight thousand (8,000) cases of eczema,[16] from private and public practice, I found that between the ages of fifteen and twenty the number of females was more than double that of men (300 to 144), whereas very early in life the males were very largely in excess, as they were also later in life; that is, during the establishment of the menses eczema is more than twice as frequent in girls than in boys of the same age. The same has been confirmed by Bohn.[10]

Instances of the influence of the menstrual function on eczema have been so frequent in my practice that I have not kept a special separate record of them, except in certain striking cases; I find, however, that in 27 patients the facts were so marked that particular note was recorded in regard to them. Their ages varied from 15 to 52 years, the greatest number in any quinquennium, six, were observed between the ages of 30 and 35.

In a number of instances the connection between the menstrual flow and the eruption was very striking, and in many of them recurrences of exacerbations of the eruption at the menstrual epoch were personally observed, and in some instances repeatedly in the same individual. In almost all of the 27 patients it was noted that the eruption improved spontaneously, immediately after the cessation of the menstrual flow. In some instances it was recorded that an eruption which had lasted off and on for years was always observed either to reappear or to be aggravated at each monthly period. The oldest patient, aged 52, still had her menses regularly, though scantily, every four weeks, with no signs of menopause. For two years she had had eczema of peculiar form on the hands, which was always greatly aggravated during menstruation, she being habitually nervous and excited before the menses, and quiet after their cessation.

Analyzing the histories of these cases I find it recorded that, in 12 patients the eruption was worse *before* the menstrual flow, in one of them a week prior to it, but generally two or three days before; in seven cases the eruption was recorded as worse *at* the menses; in five cases the eruption improved when the monthly sickness appeared; and in four cases the eruption occurred *during* the menstrual flow; in one case the eruption was worse *before* and *after* the menses; in one case it was worse two or three days *after* the discharge; and in two cases the eruption was *better* during the menses.

The location of the eczema varied greatly, almost every part of the body being affected, in different cases; in eleven patients the eruption was on the hands, and in ten on the face.

3. Herpes. Probably the next most frequent eruption having relation to the menstrual function is herpes, as so many writers dwell upon the subject. Bergh[7] states that "herpes is undoubtedly the most frequent menstrual eruption," saying that "there are women in whom almost every menstruation is accompanied with a herpes in the genital region." Among 877 cases of genital herpes recorded in the Copenhagen Hospital, between 1866 and 1889, 644, or over 73 per cent. were menstrual. In some patients, who had been long in the Hospital, the eruption was observed with each return of the menses, while others expressly stated that it recurred with almost every menstruation.

Diday and Doyon[21] are equally positive, and state that "with certain persons the return of the menstrual flow is always preceded by a little vesicular or papulo-vesicular eruption."

Unna[119] is likewise very strong in his assertions of the menstrual relations of herpes, and speaks of "habitual menstrual herpes." In the syphilitic department of the Hamburg General Hospital there were seen in four years, from 1878 to 1881, 423 cases of genital herpes in women, and, although no special cases are given, Unna speaks of prostitutes who have herpes every time they menstruate.

Legendre[77] says, "it thus happens that some women are attacked, one or two days prior to every menstruation by an eruption of herpes," and Bruneau[14] states that "the herpetic eruption frequently coincides with every menstrual epoch, whence the name, *bouton de regle*, which has been given to it." Engelmann[89] reports the case of a mother of several children who had labial herpes with each menstruation, which ceased two months after successful treatment of several uterine morbid conditions.

Further reference to literature in the direction of genital menstrual herpes is unnecessary, but it is interesting to note that little or no mention of the connection under consideration is found in the text books either on dermatology or gynæcology, and the eruption seems to be rather rare in ordinary dermatological clinics.[51] The explanation is probably found in the fact that the experience and statistics mentioned were drawn from Hospitals devoted to the reception of public women, submitted to frequent medical and police inspection.

But menstrual herpes is also of not very infrequent

occurrence in other locations. Janowsky and Schwing[66] give the case of an unmarried female, aged 30, with dysmenorrhœa, in whom an herpetic eruption appeared on the palmar surface of the left hand and sides of the fingers, with great burning and itching of both hands, in connection with the menstrual epoch, on four occasions.

Laussedat[76] reports a case where an herpetic eruption, covering several inches in the sacro-lumbar region, had recurred with each menstrual period for five years, with the single interruption of three months, during bronchitis from grip.

Chausit[21] has described, under the name herpes phlyctenodes, a recurrent vesicular eruption, in a girl aged 21, in whom the menstrual element was well marked; the eruption was commonly on the back of the hands, but occasionally on the arms, legs, and chest. Brocq,[18] in commenting on the case, says, "the menstrual troubles seemed, in this case, to coincide with the eruptive phenomena, and, so to speak, to govern them." The eruption ceased with the full establishment of the menses.

The most frequent location for the herpes of menstruation (next to the genital region) is that around the mouth, where, as Danlos[27] states, "in many women it appears regularly at each period. In most women who are thus affected the eruption is confined to a few patches at the free border of the lips; but sometimes it is more extensive, and the herpetic patches are found also on the cheeks and nose." Duhring and Hartzell[34] confirm this, stating that "in some women herpetic eruptions on the lips coincide with each menstrual period," and other writers mention it in a general way. Thus Engelmann[39] states that he has repeatedly seen herpes, especially on the lips and on the vulva, coming on two or three days before the appearance of the flow and passing away with its cessation.

This eruption of herpes about the lips in connection with menstruation I have observed many times, but find only two cases entered in the book of record referred to. One was in a young lady, aged 21, with acne, in whom there was more or less irregular, scanty, and painful menstruation. For three successive periods she had an eruption of herpes about the mouth, and had repeatedly before noticed the same, either just before or following the menstrual epoch. The other case was in a girl of 26, with stubborn eczema in both axillæ, which had lasted three years before coming under treatment. The menses were regular, every four weeks, but with much pain the first day, and for many years she would have herpes of the lips, often and only at each menstrual epoch.

Very many other diseases of the skin have been recorded, or casually mentioned, as connected with or influenced by the menstrual function, and it is difficult to arrange them further in the order of their relative frequency; mention will be made of them in perhaps their relative importance, or, in some instances, according to their pathological relations.

4. **Pemphigus.** Closely allied with herpes menstrualis is what has been described as pemphigus menstrualis by Süsemihl,[108] in the case of a girl aged eighteen. In her sixteenth year there were signs of approaching menstruation, but the menses did not appear. There appeared, however, a pretty general eruption of bullæ on the neck, chest, upper abdomen, and arms, accompanied with severe lumbar pains and many nervous phenomena; some of the bullæ were the size of a goose-egg. This eruption was repeated every four weeks, for two years, with two interruptions of three months each, and ceased with the establishment of the menses.

Grecken[49] mentions a case of a girl, aged 23, whose menstruation was regular from 14 to 20 years of age, when she had a severe shock and the menses were profuse thereafter. The eruption, which was at its height on the third day of menstruation, consisted of large and small bullæ, with milky, turbid contents, on the inner surface of both thighs and labia. The eruption had about gone on the fifth day after the menses, but returned with menstruation two months later.

Duncan[37] reports the case of a young lady, aged 25, whose regular menstruation was checked by exposure to damp and cold, and in whom a bullous eruption developed on both hands, along the course of the median and ulnar nerves, with much swelling and œdema; some of the bullæ were half an inch in diameter. One month later the menses were arrested on the second day by cold, and the eruption reappeared in the same situations, though less severe. The third menstruation was accompanied only with a hot and painful condition of the hands. Later monthly periods were normal, with no eruption.

Hardy[56] describes much the same eruption under the title *"pemphigus virginum,"* of which he had seen four cases in girls from 14 to 20 years of age. In them the menses had been irregular, and erythematous patches developed on various parts of the body, with vesico-bullæ. In two of the cases the eruption ceased with the return of regular menstruation, the other two cases were lost sight of.

Tommasoli[115] reports two cases with the same title. A girl, aged 18, menstruating from the age of 12, very abundantly for eight days, after being chilled suffered severe abdominal pain and severe general symptoms at each monthly flow, which often made her take to bed. An eruption appeared on the breast and arms, consisting of diffuse, itchy, red blotches, with subsequent vesicles and bullæ, followed by pigmented patches; lesions also appeared in the mouth and on the tongue. The eruption lasted from October, 1892, to May, 1893, with marked and constant exacerbations at each return of the menses. The second case was in a girl aged 23, in whom after grave nervous depression, an erythemato-vesicular and bullous eruption began on the left arm and invaded the other arm, limbs and all the body, with great itching. The menses were irregular, and with each return of menstruation the eruption was greatly increased.

Du Mesnil de Rochemont[26] records the case of a young girl, aged 16, with profuse and prolonged menstruation, often accompanied by pain, malaise, and vomiting, who developed on the face and extremities, and occasionally on the trunk, an eruption which he describes as pemphigus, but which corresponds more to that next to be described, dermatitis herpetiformis. The affected areas were painful during menstruation. Later she had amenorrhœa for six weeks, and during the last weeks a recurrence of a severe herpetic eruption on the face and elsewhere. Rayer[27] also confirms the influence of menstruation in the development of pemphigus.

Cummings[25] reports the case of an hysterical woman, approaching the menopause, already suffering from its advent in many ways, who had been latterly attacked again and again by severe pemphigus.

5. **Dermatitis Herpetiformis.**   Again closely allied with the two eruptions last mentioned is dermatitis herpetiformis, which may present so many different phases.

Duhring[35] has reported a case, in a woman aged 28, where the eruption, beginning in the third month of pregnancy continued for three years; with a very severe outbreak of vesicles and blebs with the arrest of menstruation, about a year later.

Brocq,[18] in his extensive study of dermatitis herpetiformis, has collected a number of instances from literature where the eruption appeared to be in relation to menstrual disturbances; he regards the case of Chausit's, already mentioned under herpes, as one of dermatitis herpetiformis, and remarks that one recognizes in many other cases the marked influence of dysmenorrhœa on successive outbreaks of the eruption.

Kerr[72] relates the case of a girl, aged 17, who while menstruating became overheated in dancing, caught cold and had a cessation of the menses, with constitutional disturbance.   Later a general eruption appeared, of pustules and blebs, ending in much desquamation. The exact nature of the eruption and its relation to the amenorrhœa do not appear very clear.

Among the cases in my book of special record before referred to, I find two of dermatitis herpetiformis, in girls aged 27 and 29, in whom the menstrual relations were often very striking. In one of them, aged 29, it is recorded that the eruption which had begun nine years before she was first seen, always developed afresh before each menstrual period. In the other case the eruption, which had lasted seven years, was always very much worse at or before menstruation, and this I observed several times while she was under treatment.

6. **Papular Eruption.** Under this very unsatisfactory diagnosis there have been reported by Schramm,[105] and also by Stiller,[107] several cases in females with dysmenorrhœa, in whom with each menstruation there appeared on various parts of the body, especially on the backs of the hands and feet, a papulo-tubercular eruption, disappearing after the cessation of the flow. On some occasions the papules developed into vesicules or pustules. In one of the cases the eruption ceased on the relief of the dysmenorrhœa. These cases could possibly be more properly classed as dermatitis herpetiformis, or as erythema multiforme. Of possibly the same nature

is the case reported by Nicolaysen[90] as a menstrual exanthem, lichen menstrualis.

7. Urticaria.   That this eruption can readily have menstrual relations is easily understood from its neurotic character, and the possibility is confirmed by the interesting observations of Scanzoni,[104] Schramm[105] and others, of its occurrence after the application of leeches to the cervix uteri.   Hebra[58] has also recorded the case of a woman with flexion of the uterus, in whom the introduction of the uterine sound produced an attack of urticaria, this having occurred fifteen times in succession.   Lawson Tait[109] reported a number of cases in which urticaria came on after abdominal section.

Hebra[59] many years ago, called attention to the connection of urticaria with disorders of the female organs, which was afterwards confirmed by Scanzoni; he also later[60] confirmed its connection with menstruation; the relation is also casually mentioned by others.

Joseph[66] relates two interesting cases in which the influence of menstruation was very striking.   Miss S., aged 29, had suffered many years from nerve disturbances, hemicrania and gastralgia; for two years she had menorrhagia and dysmenorrhœa, had a poor appetite, nausea, and was constipated, all of which troubles increased just before menstruation, which lasted three or four days.   With each menstrual flow she had urticaria, which was seldom noticed during the intervals. Under hydrotherapy and massage the menstrual troubles ceased and with them the urticaria. Mrs. S., aged 24, married 7 years, had four children, the last one two years previous to the first visit. Since then the patient had suffered much from urticaria, especially marked at the menstrual epochs. Menstruation occurred every four and a half weeks, lasted six days and was profuse; the uterus was retroflexed, large and but little movable.

Goutry[46] states that urticaria frequently appears under the influence of menstruation and gives an unpublished case, by Paul Raymond. The woman, aged 35, who had regular but scanty menstruation, suffered for a year with a periodic urticaria, coinciding with the menstrual epochs. The eruption appeared eight days before the courses, and ceased when the menstrual flow appeared.

He also cites a case by Vidal, under the name giant urticaria, coming on at the menstrual epoch, in a woman aged 26; there was a single lesion on the abdomen, oval, three by five inches in diameter, raised and œdematous. This would appear to belong rather to the next group.

Rohe[100] briefly mentions the case of a neurotic girl of 18, who suffered from an intense outbreak of ur-

ticaria at each menstrual period, although milder attacks also occurred in the intervals.

I find two cases of urticaria in my book of record,
one of them with unusual menstrual relations; this
one was in the person of a remarkably intelligent
woman, aged 50, who suffered greatly from eczema.
She stated that as a child she was exceedingly subject
to urticaria, especially at the grape season, but when
the menses appeared the tendency ceased entirely, and
she had not suffered therefrom since. In the other
case, a married woman of 27, urticaria appeared on
two occasions two days before the menses, and ceased
the day after they were finished.

8. **Œdema and Cutaneous Nodes.** Closely
related to urticaria are the cases of acute circumscribed œdema of Quincke,[95] and other forms of cutaneous swelling, and Börner[12] has reported three
cases where such were clearly connected with menstruation; Quincke also noticed the relationship. Börner says, "In women, both menstruation and the cli-
macteric, with the nervous disturbances known to ac-
company them, and with attendant loss of blood,
would furnish a predisposition to such swellings,
which are at times solely associated with such
epochs." In one girl, aged 15, the following conditions were noted on each of the four months preceding her visit. "On the day before menstruation, as

well as on the first three days of the period, œdema appears on the forehead, in circumscribed bumps, as if stung by an insect. This condition also appears as a more uniform swelling on the cheeks and temples." In the case of another girl, aged 15½, who had menstruated two years, an œdematous swelling over the bridge of the nose began one week before menstruation. This phenomenon lasted until the third day of the period, when it disappeared; the maximum seemed to be on the day the menses came. In a third case the œdema appeared in the lower eyelids, upper lip, palms of hands, knees, malleoli and soles of the feet.

McGillicuddy[62] records the case of a young lady, aged 20, with extremely painful menstruation, who had, with each period, swelling of the left foot and leg, and also of the face. He says, "I have seen her face much distorted on these occasions by œdema around the eyes and at the base of the nose."

DeKeyser[28] presented a patient at the Belgium Dermatological Society with a condition of angio-neurotic œdema simulating erysipelas. The girl was aged 21, and for two years had had an attack each month, at the monthly period, which was natural. The swelling extended from the eyebrows to the line of the mouth, and was red and shiny, with occasional vesicles about the upper lip and eyebrows; it lasted a week and disappeared spontaneously, with no fever. He mentioned another case in a girl who had never menstruated, and who at the age of 17 began to suffer each month with an erysipelatous œdema of the face. This was accompanied with deep pains in the lower abdomen, similar to those often attending menstruation; on examination there was only a slight endometritis.

Hobbs[62] reports the case of an unmarried woman aged 39, who for 15 years had suffered from very severe migraine, with the menstrual periods. Eleven years previous to her first visit she had begun to notice, with each menstruation, a thickening in the left frontal region, moving with the skin; it was oval, three by one inches in diameter, and disappeared entirely with the headache, without leaving a trace. The next menstrual epoch it reappeared, with others, and sometimes she would have a dozen or more on the head, later also on the fingers and then on the right knee. Subsequently she developed rheumatic pains.

Engelmann[39] mentions two cases where there were small tumefactions on the forehead, breast and back, which appeared at the time of menstrual congestion, passing away with the cessation of the menstrual flow as rapidly as they had come. The patients were the subjects of uterine disease and suffered from many other reflex symptoms.

I have had one remarkable case of angio-neurotic œdema, in a widow aged 40, where the influence of menstruation was very clearly shown several times. While the trouble had lasted off and on for 16 years, beginning two months after the death of her husband, she would often be free from it for some time, when it would suddenly burst out a day or two before menstruation, as I observed several times, lasting about until the cessation of the menses. The swellings generally appeared on the face, but sometimes affected also the extremities.

In another case, in a young lady, aged 24, there was frequently swelling about the eyes and lips with each menstrual period.

9. **Erythema.** Again closely allied to the forms of angio-neurotic disturbance of the cutaneous circulation already mentioned are the varieties of erythema simplex, multiforme, and nodosum, which have been repeatedly observed in connection with menstruation, and are thus casually mentioned by many writers. Polotebnoff[94] in his exhaustive study of the disease says, "Menstruation has, undoubtedly, a marked influence upon the production of erythema."

The milder form of erythema simplex, more or less transient, recurrent at each menstruation, is familiar to all, and has seldom been reported upon.

Behrend[5] mentions the case of a woman aged 30, who with each menstruation had a diffuse, hyperæmic erythema of the whole face, which began shortly before the flow and faded with its cessation.

Engelmann[39] records several cases of erythema of the face which yielded to careful local uterine treatment; in one of them the condition was greatly aggravated during menstruation. He also quotes Kidd[78] as recording a striking case of erythema uterinum.

McGillicuddy[82] records the case of a girl, aged 20, who had unilateral flushing of the face, coming on from three to eight days before each menstrual epoch, and which disappeared as the flow came on; and another of a married woman, aged 40, where, with menstruation every two weeks, there was a swelling of the abdomen, which became of a dark or bluish-red color, with congestion and redness of the face. He also cites a case by Weir Mitchell somewhat similar, in a young married woman with irregular menses, who at menstruation had abdominal swelling, with skin tense and red.

Edebohls[38] has reported the case of a girl aged 19, who presented a peculiar erythematous eruption on the right side of the face, from the middle of the temple to near the angle of the jaw. The eruption had appeared regularly two days before the men-

strual flow, fading with its cessation; this had occurred for three years, from 15 to 18 years of age,
with then an interruption of nine months, when it
again recurred regularly each month. She suffered
from severe dysmenorrhœa, for which she was cu-
retted, when the eruption ceased for three months.
Double ovarian disease was then discovered and the
organs were removed, but the eruption "reappeared
with clock-like regularity once a month," and rather
more intensely.

Danlos[27] cites a case, exhibited by Lallier, where
for eight months a woman had an erythema multiforme on the back of the hands, with each menstruation, it disappearing in the time between. The
woman was in good health and the menstruation regular.

Goutry[48] reports an interesting case of erythema
multiforme in an emotional woman aged 34 years,
whose menses were regular, every twenty days. The
eruption, which was located mainly on the backs of
the hands, first appeared at the age of 16, a few
months before the establishment of the menses, new
lesions coming out with each subsequent menstruation. Married at 21, the eruption ceased during
pregnancy, but reappeared with the menses, until arrested by the next pregnancy, when it again recurred
a few days before or with each menstruation. She

was also constipated, and noticed that when this constipation was aggravated she had more eruption.

Stiller[107] describes a very characteristic erythema multiforme, with ring-shaped and gyrate lesions, in a woman of 30, who had long suffered from amenorrhœa, the menses seldom appearing oftener than from six to ten weeks.   When there was much delay there appeared lesions on the backs of the hands and forearms, more rarely on the lower limbs; with the onset of the menses the eruption paled and flattened, reappearing in five or six weeks, if the menses did not appear.   There was no disease of the sexual organs except a slight catarrh.

Laredde[75] presented at the French Dermatological Society a woman, aged 33, who for nearly twenty years had had certain eruptions recurrent at almost every menstrual period.   Upon the face the eruption was herpetic, but on the hands there were papules and patches of erythema multiforme, and on the legs occasional purpuric lesions.   It is more than probable that the cases already mentioned under "papular eruption" (6) were of this nature.

Gerson[45] presented a woman, aged 42, at the Berlin Dermatological Society, with a vesicating erythema occurring only when exposed to heat, which he thought partly due to dysmenorrhœa, which had lasted since puberty; but the connection between the two appeared very improbable to the members present.

Hardy[55] is frequently quoted as regarding menstrual disturbances a frequent cause of erythema nodosum, but I have been unable to find more than a brief mention of the same.

Goutry reports a case by Genet[44] in which erythema nodosum appeared on the lower extremities two days after the suppression of the menses.

Among my own recorded cases I find a number in whom erythema simplex was strikingly displayed, especially on the face, in connection with menstruation. In one case, a lady aged 36, mother of four children, the face has been intensely red much of the time, as a result of chronic uterine trouble since her last confinement, some three years ago; the congestion has improved when she has submitted to gynæcological treatment. Time and again she has noticed the great aggravation of the redness and burning one or two days before the menstrual period, and its subsidence on the second day of the flow, and the same was personally observed on a number of occasions. In another case, that of a married lady aged 34, with one child, aged 10, and no other pregnancies, the erythema of the face was always immensely aggravated just before menstruation, which was irregular. She had also digestive and urinary disturbances, and when these were rectified medically the aggravation was not noticed at the menstrual period. In another case, that of a lady aged 23, an erythema simplex began during pregnancy, seven years before, and disappeared upon miscarriage. It then returned and was observed to be always worse before and after each menstruation. A young lady, aged 23, has for several years had great erythematous flushing of the face with each menstruation, it subsiding when the flow was over. The menses are regular, every four weeks, lasting five days, generally with some, but not severe, pain.

A case of erythema multiforme was observed in a lady aged 35, who had had a number of attacks during the preceding three years, mainly on the fingers and hands; the eruption appeared or was markedly worse always before or during menstruation, and improved spontaneously when it was past. The menses were regular and painless, every twenty-six to twenty-eight days, and lasted five or six days, which was about the duration of each attack. She was a neurotic subject, always more or less depressed by work and worry.

10. Erysipelas. So many writers mention the connection of true erysipelas with menstruation, and the number of separately reported cases is so large, that the relationship must be accepted as a fact;

Thomas, Godot, Tourneux, Cachera, and Salvy have written extensive theses on the subject. But in the light of what has preceded it is readily understood that certain of the cases of so-called "menstrual erysipelas" may belong more properly to some of the conditions already mentioned.

Thomas,[118] the first to write fully on this subject, in 1875, collected in his thesis thirteen cases, one personal, in seven of which "the erysipelas recurred punctually at each menstrual epoch, respectively two, three, four, five, seven, twelve, and thirty-five times; in another case, lasting five years, there were about fifty attacks, interrupted by gestation.

Godot[47] gives the histories of twelve cases (some of them already quoted by Thomas) one of the patients having had five attacks, another twelve, and others had had repeated attacks at the menstrual period.

Tourneux[116] in 1886, who recognizes the microbic nature of erysipelas, gives a very interesting study of the subject, detailing five cases, four of them already quoted in the above.

Cachera[19] in 1891, made a further careful study of menstrual erysipelas, from a bacteriological standpoint, and gives twelve cases, five of them previously unpublished. In one of them the streptococcus, with also staphylococcus albus, were demonstrated; there were several recurrences at the menstrual period, in one of which the temperature rose to 104°. In another case "the microbes characteristic of erysipelas" were also found.

Salvy[102] has made a very interesting and careful review of menstrual erysipelas, with bibliography and analysis of preceding observations, with many of his own. He gives details of sixteen cases in which there were menstrual relations, often of a very decided and striking character; the patients ranged from twenty to forty-nine years of age. In all the cases there was a preceding chill, and constitutional symptoms, with elevation of temperature, in many 104° F. and over with acceleration of the pulse up to 116. In six cases there were recurrences a number of times with the menses, and he quotes Roger[94] in regard to a case in a woman who had thus had forty-six recurrences.

The course of menstrual erysipelas is generally mild, and according to Salvy the disease does not seem to affect the menstruation, nor does the latter affect the erysipelas greatly, except that it tends to cease with the development of the menses. He thinks it is less frequent than commonly supposed, and among 323 cases of erysipelas observed by Roger there were thirteen of menstrual erysipelas; and of 487 of his own cases, there were twenty-eight showing this relationship, a total of forty-one cases in 810, or 5.20 per cent.

Behrend[5] mentions the case of a girl, where he personally observed erysipelas three or four times, always at the time of the menses, with considerable elevation of temperature, which disappeared completely thereafter. Neligan[89] reported a very characteristic erysipelas in a girl, beginning and ending with each menstruation for a long time.

Danlos[27] gives and cites a number of cases, some of which, at least, appear to have been unquestionably true erysipelas.

Wagner[121] has reported three cases, in one of whom the temperature was 104°.2 F.; Pauli[92] one in which it reached almost 105° F.; and Batuand[4] one in which it was about 104° F. In one of Wagner's cases, a girl of 16, who had menstruated regularly from her fourteenth year, it is stated that "from the first appearance of menstruation, four or five days before the period, a facial erysipelas would appear, lasting about eight days. At first it involved the face only, later the scalp was invaded, causing loss of hair."

Grelletty[52] gives two cases, in one of which, in a girl aged 21, the menses were usually retarded and nearly always preceded by an eruption of erysipelas, which he describes very clearly; on the establishment of the menstrual flow all symptoms subsided. The same also happened in a second case, in a woman aged 37 years.

Deligny[29] in studying the alterations of the skin which are produced at the time of puberty and at the menopause, writes as follows: "Many authors have cited cases of erysipelas at the moment of menstrual cessation. Tissot reports a case in which erysipelas occurred fifteen times during the two years succeeding the menopause. Behier observed a woman of 54 in whom the monthly flow was replaced at correspondingly regular intervals by erysipelas of the face. Numerous cases have also been reported at the time of puberty."

Many authors, especially the French, mention the connection very positively, and Rayer[97] states that "in amenorrhœa erysipelas sometimes recurs periodically at the time at which menstruation should take place."

Massalongo[84] reports a singular case in which a girl, aged 22, had sixty recurrences of erysipelas with menstruation. When 16 years of age she had a severe attack of facial erysipelas, which lasted, with several relapses, for some months. At about 17½ years of age the first menstruation appeared, preceded by intense headache and general malaise. On the second day of the flow she had facial erysipelas, with fever and constitutional symptoms. Four days later,

as the menses ceased, the fever went down, and the
eruption subsided, with desquamation. From that
time on for sixty months the girl had regularly an
attack of facial erysipelas, with each menstrual flow,
appearing from the first to the third day of the period. She never had a menstrual period without an
attack of erysipelas, and with the exception of the
first attack she never suffered from erysipelas except
at the menstrual epoch.

The rationale of the connection of erysipelas with
menstruation will be considered later, in connection
with the discussion of the general influences operat-
ing to cause the relations under consideration.

11. Ecchymoses and Purpura. The frequent
general disturbances of the circulation during the
menstrual period, with the many neurotic phenomena liable to occur, make it easy to understand how changes can take place in the capillaries
leading to ecchymoses and purpura. Stiller[107] records the case of a well-nourished but somewhat anæmic woman, aged 27, whose menses were normal
in time and duration, though sometimes a little scanty,
who presented the following condition: For a year
and a half, a few days before each menstruation,
there appeared on the chin, lower part of the cheeks,
and upper lip, bluish irregular spots, about the size
of the nail, which did not disappear on pressure and

were accompanied with no unpleasant sensation. On cessation of the flow the spots turned yellow and disappeared.

Wilhelm[128] has reported the case of a healthy woman, aged 29, with regular and almost painless menstruation, who for about five years suffered from a menstrual eruption. Two or three days before the beginning of menstruation she noticed small, dark red elevations, often growing as large as a walnut, and disappearing with the cessation of the menses. These were commonly seated on the thighs, occasionally on the lower legs: there was one large sub-cutaneous hémorrhage in the left popliteal space. These ecchymoses disappeared in a few days, the smaller leaving almost no trace, the larger a yellowish stain. These appearances came regularly with menstruation, but did not occur when the' latter was interrupted by pregnancy and lactation.

Parvin[91] reported as vicarious menstruation, a case which may be classed in this group. She was a girl, who menstruated normally from the age of 14 to that of 16, when she was admitted to the Reformatory, delicate and anæmic. The menses then ceased for six months, and then there occurred a purplish swelling of both lips, especially the lower, so marked as to suggest impending gangrenous inflammation: a little blood oozed from the inner surface of the lower lip. In four days all hemorrhage ceased, and the lips resumed a normal size and color. The same phenomena recurred three times, subsequently, at monthly intervals.

Townsend[117] reports the case of a girl aged 13, with a tendency to hæmophilia who exhibited pale red ecchymoses on the shoulders and elbows at the first menstruation.

Danlos[27] cites several cases of purpura and hemorrhagic conditions of the skin in connection with menstruation.

Rohe[100] refers to a case, reported by a friend, "in which a purpuric eruption appeared on the lower extremities every month, while the menstrual flow was arrested."

In the discussion of Edebohl's case, referred to under erythema (9), Currier[26] stated that he had under his observation a case with a similar history, but the eruption resembled purpura.

Goutry quotes Morin[86] in regard to a woman aged 33, in whom purpura recurred on the extremities with each menstruation. She was married at 19 and had two children, the latter at 23 years of age. Six or seven months after the birth of the last child she began to have purpuric spots on the arms and legs which appeared commonly two or three days before the flow, more rarely with it: in twenty-four hours the eruption reached its height, and disappeared in eight to ten days.

Leveque[78] reports the case of a neurotic woman, aged 46, in whom a purpura urticans developed, first on the lower extremities, following or with the occurrence of the menses before their time, in consequence of a prolonged fit of anger. The menses were always very regular, and she had never previously had any affection of the skin.

In this connection should be noticed the cases of so-called "bloody sweat" and hemorrhage from skin lesions, of which a number of instances have been recorded where the menstrual relations were most pronounced. McCall Anderson[2] has reported a very interesting case, and collected material bearing on the subject. In most of the reported cases of "bloody sweat" the bleeding has been from erythematous or other lesions, which form spontaneously on various parts of the body, but the evidence is very conclusive that the hemorrhage has occurred either with or in place of the menstrual flow.

Royer Collard[101] is quoted by Goutry in regard to a case which appears to be of this character. A young Norwegian girl, at the time of her first menstrual epoch suddenly found her body covered with large and very red blotches, especially marked about the breasts: at the same time she had severe headache

and toochache. Sudorifics were given, which produced a very abundant bloody sweat from the lesions.
The blotches and other symptoms disappeared soon,
but returned with the next menstrual period.

Clairborne[22] observed the case of a pale, poorly-
nourished girl, of 16, who began to menstruate at 13,
and in whom, every month, two or three days before
the period, a red spot appeared under each eye. The
skin became red, blood rose to the surface and oozed
through, forming a clot which dried to a crust. This
lasted through the period and then disappeared spontaneously. A somewhat similar case has been reported by Dolganoff.[32]

The subject of vicarious menstruation is a large
one, and many authentic cases are found in literature
of monthly hemorrhages from different organs. Cases
of bleeding from ulcers at the menstrual epoch are
reported by Coughlin,[24] Green,[50] Kelsey,[71] Moses,[87]
Tedrowe,[110] Tyrrell,[118] and others, also from a facial
nævus by Bloom.[9]

12. Pruritus. It is not at all uncommon to
find an increased pruritus at the menstrual epoch, in
connection with many diseases of the skin, and occasionally this symptom will be very distressing at this
time. In certain instances pruritus exists as a disease, an impairment of innervation, whose only sign
is the itching, and whose only lesions are those which

are the result of scratching, or from measures employed to give relief. In some of these cases the cutaneous irritation is manifested only at the time of menstruation, and in others it is immensely aggravated at this period.

Danlos[27] cites a case of violent general itching following the suppression of the menses, in a woman aged 36; the back and shoulders were principally affected.

Deligny[30] reports a case of pruritus vulvæ, where a quite intense and constant itching preceded the menstrual flow by some four or five days. All symptoms disappeared as soon as the flow began.

Many writers speak of pruritus as an accompaniment of the menopause, and with derangement of the sexual organs, and some casually allude to it as a regular occurrence at the menstrual period, in rare cases.

Dubreuilh[38] mentions that, in a case of parapsoriasis, in a woman aged 40, "at the moment of menstruation the pruritus becomes intense, and at the same time the eruption becomes more red."

In my book of notes, already referred to, I find mention of eight cases of pruritus in which record is made in regard to the influence of the menstrual function, in this state, in females aged respectively 30, 35, 35, 36, 38, 40, 44, 50; the first three and the sev-

enth were single, the last three and the eighth married. In one of them, single, aged 35, the pruritus,
which was more or less general, began two days before each flow, and ceased abruptly when menstruation occurred; the case was under observation for over
a year, and this was repeatedly noticed. The two
nights before the period were often quite sleepless
from the itching; the menses were regular and normal, every four weeks.

In four other cases of more or less general pruritus, the itching was markedly worse just before and
during menstruation, while in a fifth case, in which
there was a history of much uterine trouble and dysmenorrhœa, it is recorded that the itching was better during the menstrual period. In another case,
in a lady aged 35, with pruritus of the vulva and
anus, it is recorded that the itching was very much
worse before and after menstruation.

13. Psoriasis and Dermatitis Seborrhœica.
One would hardly expect that such eruptions as these
would be affected by the menstruation, but many
writers speak of psoriasis being greatly aggravated
at that time, with itching, as in the case of parapsoriasis by Dubreuilh,[13] mentioned in the last section. Danlos[17] cites a rather doubtful case in a
woman aged 36, who had had psoriasis eight years,
in whom the menses, always irregular, gradually

ceased during this period; and he attributes the early cessation to be due to the influence of the prolonged eruption!

I have repeatedly observed the influence of menstruation on psoriasis, causing increased development of new lesions, and congestion and aggravation of old patches, often with much itching, just before or during the menstrual flow. In two cases, married women, aged 30 and 42, these features were so striking as to cause special mention to be made in the book of record already referred to.

In three cases of dermatitis seborrhœica I find that special record was made of menstrual relations. In one young lady, aged 29, it was recorded that the eruption was worse just before the menses, and decidedly better after it was over: while in two other cases, a girl of 19 and a woman of 44, the eruption was better at the time of menstruation, and in the last case it was recorded that it almost disappeared at some menstrual periods.

14. Hyperidrosis. The occurrence of sweating, general or localized, in connection with menstruation or with uterine relations, is a well-recognized fact, mentioned by many writers.

Deligny[80] dwells upon the subject and mentions a number of interesting cases, some of which may be referred to. In one instance, a woman, for eleven years, had cold sweats, localized about the waist, abdomen, and thighs, coming on regularly each month. He quotes a somewhat similar case by Levy, where a woman, aged 28, had a local perspiration of the chest at the beginning of each menstrual epoch. In the case of a young girl, of 13, with painful menstruation, there were, at each menstrual period, flashes of heat followed by abundant perspiration of the head and face. In another girl, aged 15, who had menstruated once and not again for a year, there was a profuse perspiration of the chest and axillæ, with a penetrating odor, and the subsequent production of a papular eczema. With the re-establishment of the menstrual flow the hyperidrosis and eczema both disappeared.

Gillet[46] narrates the case of a married woman, aged 35, who had menstruated regularly from the age of 14, and in whom, five months previous to the report, the menses had ceased without known cause. During this time abundant sweating had occurred, from insignificant causes, at periods corresponding to the absent menses: in the interval the sweating was very slight. Under appropriate treatment the menses reappeared, and the sweating ceased entirely.

The occurrence of abundant perspiration in connection with the menopause is well known to all.

Tilt[114] records perspirations as occurring in 290 out of 500 women at the change of life.

Liégeois[80] has made a careful study of sweating occurring with the menopause, citing many authorities and giving a number of personal cases.

Bromidrosis, or offensive sweating, is also occasionally met with in connection with menstruation. Cazal[20] speaks of certain women who, at the time of menstruation, have abundant perspiration, with special odor. Others also mention the subject casually, but I can find no recorded cases and have no marked personal instances to record.

15. **Chloasma and Melanoderma.** The pigmentary changes in the skin which are associated with diseases of the female sexual organs and pregnancy are well known, and need not occupy us here; except to state that certain writers attribute the pigmentary deposit to absence of the menstrual flow. Some of the cases which have been thus reported, and also certain of those in connection with menstruation, appear to be instances of feigned eruption, and some have been proved to be self-produced by means of various pigmentary substances.

But there is also abundant evidence that in some instances a pigmentary deposit may occur in the skin in connection with menstruation, to which various

names, such as chloasma uterinum, melasma, melanoderma, cyanopathy, etc., have been given.

Banks[2] has collected from a number of writers,
Yonge,[120] Teevan,[111] Neligan,[89] and others, a vari-
ety of cases exhibiting changes in the color of the
skin in connection with derangement or suppression
of menstruation, which are worthy of attention, although writers have discredited some of them as
possibly being self-produced. He also gives a personal case, in a girl, aged 23, who had irregular cata-
menia, with amenorrhœa, in which there was vicarious
menstruation in the way of periodical hæmoptysis.
She presented a remarkable discoloration about the
eyes, especially beneath them, which was more vivid
during the three or four days of hæmoptysis each
month.

Billard[6] reports a remarkable case, in a girl aged
16, who had menstruated two years, who had a blue
discoloration on the skin, beginning slightly about
the eyes with her first menstruation. This
increased with each menstrual flow, until when first
seen the face, neck, and upper part of the chest were
affected; when the period was past the coloration
largely faded. The menses were regular, but at each
occurrence she had a stuffed-up feeling, and a cough
with bloody sputa, and later hæmatemesis.

Leroy de Mericourt[70] reported three cases in which

brown discoloration appeared on the eyelids, following suppression of the menses, and in one case the color was blue.

Goutry[48] has reported the case of a woman, aged 29, with a chloasmic discoloration on the forehead and cheeks, like that of pregnancy, but who had never conceived. Her menses were irregular and scanty, and the pigmentation increased and extended for four or five days at that time, the skin remaining a little colored between.

Many writers mention incidentally the tendency to cutaneous pigmentation in connection with menstrual irregularities. Thus Rohe[100] says, "Localized increase of the cutaneous pigment is one of the most frequent accompaniments of derangement of the generative apparatus in the female. The surface usually affected is the face, although in some cases reported the entire body has showed a marked discoloration. * * * The patches are yellowish-brown to dark brown in color, and are most frequently found on the forehead, cheeks and eyelids. * * * Women subject to menstrual irregularities are especially prone to this pigmentary hypertrophy."

Guibout[54] mentions chloasma as associated with metrorrhagia. Erasmus Wilson[125] reports a pigmented patch appearing on the front of the neck of a young lady following the sudden suppression of

menstruation. Alibert[1] noted the occurrence of ephelides or chloasma in young girls whose menstruation
was arrested. Grelletty[53] says that there are women
who are troubled with ephelides only at the time of
menstruation.

Engelmann[39] recognizes fully the association between pigmentation of the skin and uterine disease,
and gives several illustrative cases: he says that "the
pigmentation of the eyelids must be distinguished
from the simple venous lividity so marked during
menstruation."

I have observed several cases, two of which were
so striking as to cause special record to be made. One
was in a widow, aged 31, whose husband died about
the time of her second confinement, six years previous to her first visit. Her chloasma of the face appeared during this second pregnancy, and had lasted
more or less ever since. Two or three days before
each menstrual epoch the eruption becomes very
much darker, and remains so until the fifth day, when
it lightens very decidedly. The other case was in a
young unmarried woman, aged 30, in whom the
chloasma always becomes very much darker two days
before the appearance of the menses, when the eyes
also become swollen.

16. **Furunculosis and Abscess.** While it may
seem irrational to suppose that the menstrual state

can affect conditions which are commonly recognized to be dependent upon the presence of a micro-organism, there is abundant evidence to be found that such is the case. The occurrence of boils and abscesses, small and large, in the vulva at the time of menstruation is familiar to all, while in acne it will be observed time and again that pustules develop at the menstrual period.

Loewenberg[81] first called attention to the subject, in his elaborate study of furunculosis, devoting a section to the relation of menstruation to the appearance of furuncles; he speaks of their occurrence in the ear, more or less regularly either before or during each catamenial period, as common enough and quite well known. He gives the case of the young wife of a physician who for three or four years invariably had furuncles of the external auditory canal toward the end of each menstrual epoch, or immediately afterward.

Recognizing fully the microbic nature of the trouble, he says: "A boil having once occurred, by introduction of the specific germ into a hair follicle, the pus which escapes may introduce permanent germs (Dauersporen) into other follicles or auricular glands. Under ordinary conditions the resisting power of the system is sufficient to keep these germs latent, but the systemic depression often accompanying the menses reduces the resisting power, and the germs become active."

Goutry[48] endorses this and cites a case from Bouchard,[11] where a woman for five or six months had furuncles at each catamenial period: the first time she had more than forty. After intestinal antisepsis the menses appeared, without any furuncles, and so recurred for several months.

Moutard-Martin[88] reports the case of a girl, who had had furuncles incessantly from the age of thirteen until the menses appeared at fifteen, when they ceased to appear. Menstruation ceased two months later, and the furuncles reappeared, and were not checked until the menses were again re-established.

I have observed the tendency to pus formation to be increased at the menstrual period, but find only two cases of furuncles in the record referred to. A lady, aged 35, had had eczema at the back of the scalp for two years previous to her first visit, accompanied with boils on various parts of the body. She had noticed the boils to appear a few days before the occurrence of menstruation, and to be better immediately after. In another lady, aged 48, with some uterine trouble, there has been often an occurrence of boils four or five days before the menses, on many occasions, on two of which I saw her: they were generally in the anal region.

I have also had one very striking case of multiple abscess of the scalp in which the menstrual relations were personally observed on a number of occasions, over a considerable period of time. The girl, aged 18, was poorly nourished, and lived in unhealthy surroundings, working at a trade. For seven or eight months she had had abscesses, of an indolent character on the scalp, and when first seen perhaps a dozen slightly elevated, purplish-red masses, of various sizes, could be discovered, with distinct fluctuation in many of them, and with some bald areas, the site of former lesions. There was no trichophytic disease, but a history of seborrhœic dermatitis. Under active treatment, internal and external, the scalp improved, but on several occasions she returned with accession of new abscesses at the time of menstruation. It was nearly a year before the tendency to the formation of abscesses was finally overcome.

17. Syphilis. This is also a disease in which it would hardly be expected that the menstrual function would exercise any influence on its lesions; but here also it may often be observed that its later manifestations on the skin are modified at the time of menstruation. This has been casually noticed by me, and also remarked on by patients, but I find only two cases entered on my special book of record. These were in women aged 29 and 44 years, with late syphilide

of the palm. They have both of them noticed repeatedly that the eruption was greatly aggravated during menstruation, as I myself have observed. The very day of this writing the second patient exhibited it most strikingly. For two or three years the menses have been getting irregular, sometimes with intervals of three months, and sometimes continuing for several weeks. The menses have now been lasting three weeks, and the right palm, which was very well, when seen three weeks ago, has during this interval been again greatly affected, and more or less inflamed, with a new area spreading continuously, she being still under active treatment.

May it not be that some of the peculiarities in the course of syphilis, noticed by many, and especially dwelt on by Fournier, are, in a measure, due to menstrual influence? It has been suggested that the monthly flow removes some of the syphilitic virus, and from the marked proneness of the product of conception to be seriously affected by the poison, we see that the latter has a great tendency towards the uterus.

18. Lupus. While lupus usually begins before the advent of menstruation, there are several observations on record showing the influence of the menstrual function on the development or character of the eruption. Vrain[120] reports two cases in which the eruption was markedly influenced at the menstrual

epochs. Goutry[48] records a case of lupus from the clinic of Fournier in Paris, where the effect of menstruation was shown in a manner contrary to that usually observed. A woman, aged 24, had had lupus of the left cheek, beginning at the age of 8 years; as soon as the menstruation appeared the eruption paled, and was said to have "disappeared," only to appear when the menses ceased. She was twice pregnant, and during this time the redness disappeared, and returned two months later.

Since my attention was called to this subject I have observed one case of lupus vulgaris, affecting the nose, upper lip and both cheeks, in which the eruption became much worse at the menopause.

I find also four cases of *lupus erythematosus* entered on my book of record, in which the effects of menstruation were marked on a number of occasions. Mrs. H., a widow, aged 29, with a very diffused eruption of five years' duration, on both sides of the face, behind the right ear, and scattered through the scalp, had noticed that the eruption was always worse at menstruation, and that new spots appeared at that time. Miss S., aged 30, had had the eruption for twelve years, it beginning on the end of the nose, and gradually appearing on various parts of the face and behind the ears. The eruption had always been irritated and inflamed during menstruation, which was profuse. Miss B., aged 38, who was under my observation for a year and a half, first noticed the eruption on the scalp twelve years before her first visit. It had been preceded by swollen glands below the ears, which suppurated and crusted every month, a week before the menses. The eruption had remained and attacked other parts of the scalp, face, and behind the ears. Her menstruation was peculiar, sometimes six days in being established, and then lasting scantily for two or three days, and was often much delayed. In January, 1894, it was recorded: "The eruption was again very much worse just before the menses, which appeared on the 24th: the ears are now inflamed and raw in places, and the spots on the scalp are inflamed and crusted. The eruption always begins to show signs of aggravation about a week before menstruation is expected, when the breasts begin to feel sore; the excitement lasts until menstruation is fairly begun, and then goes down rapidly. Two weeks ago, when last here, there was almost no eruption visible, there are now a considerable number of new spots, on the face and behind the ears, and all feel hot and burning." The same conditions had been observed and recorded by me in connection with previous menstrual periods. Mrs. T., aged 43, with one child, aged 8, had long suffered with painful menstruation, and had much leucorrhœa and backache from uterine version and laceration, and had developed lupus erythematosus three years previous to her first visit, in 1884; she was seen at intervals for twelve years thereafter, and the effects of menstruation were frequently noted. At one time the eruption almost entirely disappeared during pregnancy, leaving only slight pink scars. The eruption during its whole course affected much of the face, also the backs of the hands, and was repeatedly noticed to be aggravated at menstruation. On January 31, 1894, it was recorded that "the eruption is always worse during and after the menstrual period, and now, at that time, there are several inflamed points in the old scars, especially in the left eyebrow and on the right side of the nose."

19. Epithelioma. Even so local a disease as epithelioma may be affected by menstruation, as I have observed in one striking case. Miss G., aged 31, had a large, ulcerating epithelioma on the right temple and cheek, which had started from an injury many years before; the surface had been vigorously treated, but had never healed, and the diseased area had gradually extended until it covered several square inches, involving the eye. It was recorded March 12, 1894, that "the diseased area was greatly inflamed, as also the eye, menstruation having begun

four days previously, and also that she had observed the same condition at previous menstruations."

20. **Scleroderma and Morphœa.** Many, years ago Thirial,[112] in first describing scleroderma, noted its connection with amenorrhœa. In one young woman, aged 31, it followed a five months' suppression, and in a girl, aged 15, it occurred shortly after suppression of the menses. In the latter case the menses returned for a day and the skin became less hard, and six months after the appearance of the disease they returned regularly, and at once the skin began to soften and the disease disappeared entirely without treatment, after the patient left the hospital. It is well known that over two-thirds of the cases of scleroderma occur in females, and in view of its probable tropho-neurotic origin it is quite likely that further observation will show other instances where menstruation had material relation to the disease.

Byers[18] has reported four cases of *Raynaud's disease* associated with diminished or arrested menstruation.

21. **Alopecia Areata.** In one patient of mine, with very generalized alopecia areata, which ultimately affected the entire scalp, eyebrows, lashes, and most of the body, there was a menstrual connection which was very striking; she was aged 26, unmarried, and had long suffered from delayed,

scanty, and painful menstruation. For four or five days before the menses appeared, and for a day or two after, she suffered intensely from itching of the scalp, which at times was almost unbearable. She suffered from a number of neuroses, and the skin had itched before the hair began to fall.

22. Hypertrichosis. Many writers have commented on the fact that superfluous hairs occur in connection with deficient or disturbed menstruation, and Jamieson[44] has particularly emphasized the fact, with cases. This I have observed in numerous instances, but as the immediate effect of menstrual disturbances was not particularly noticed, I had not entered the cases on the book of record referred to. The well-known observation of superfluous hairs, especially on the chin after the menopause, corroborates the fact of menstrual relations in this condition.

On my book of record I find mention of several other skin conditions, with menstrual relations, which can hardly be classified with the preceding observations.

A lady, aged 43, had an inflammation on the radial side of the right thumb, which she said that she had noticed every month, for seven or eight years, in connection with menstruation. It always occurred about two or three days before the flow, and disappeared soon after; she could always predict the menses in two or three days by the condition of the thumb. Two months later the same condition was again personally observed. She said that when she was in the tropics this did not occur.

A young lady, aged 16, who had had eczema in infancy, exhibited a hard, dry, cracked condition about the tips of the fingers, and around the nails for five or six years. Since the appearance of the menses, which began at 12, and were apt to be a week or so late, she had noticed that the affected parts were always worse, swelling and cracking, just before the monthly period.

A young lady, aged 24, whose menses were always irregular, up to six weeks, lasting two days, and not very painful, exhibited time and again lesions on the skin of a peculiar character with each menstrual flow. While they were frequently acne-form in appearance they presented often deep, shot-like lesions which would remain a long time, often suppurating slightly, and leave a pigmented stain, with perhaps superficial cicatrix. They came frequently on the face or neck, but also on the backs of the hands and forearms, and were regarded as hydradenitis suppurativa. She was under observation for eighteen months, and their development or increase just before the menstrual flow was observed on a number of occasions.

CHAPTER III.

ANALYSIS OF FACTS AND THEORIES.

Many theories have been put forth to explain the nature and causes of the various functional and other derangements occurring in different organs in connection with menstruation. It would be useless to discuss them all here, as many of them relate to former times, before the days of exact observation. The most plausible seem to be the three outlined in the opening chapter, namely:

1. That of *"Cyclic Changes" taking place in the general system:*

2. *Auto-intoxication of genital origin:*

3. *Nervous reflex irritation from the congested condition of the uterus and ovaries.*

These we will consider in turn, and shall find that the first and third are well based and have reasonable support: the second is somewhat problematical, and more light is needed on this, as indeed on all hypotheses as to the actual cause of the clinical phenomena which have been recorded by many observers.

However difficult it may be to understand, the fact

remains that, in many scores of cases, relating to over a score of diseased conditions of the skin, which have been observed and recorded by several scores of trained and careful clinicians, there have occurred changes in the skin having close relationship to the monthly menstrual flow: and there must be some reason for the phenomena in question.

It will be seen that the diseases of the skin already mentioned with menstrual relations are of very varied character, and represent almost all the groups known to dermatology: and it is likely that when attention is directed more to this subject others may be added to the list already given. Thus, the *congestive* and *inflammatory* dermatoses are represented by eczema, herpes, pemphigus, dermatitis herpetiformis, and others, to the number of ten in all: *glandular diseases* by acne and hyperidrosis: *neurotic* affections by pruritus, and perhaps others: *hypertrophic* conditions by chloasma, scleroderma, and hypertrichosis: *atrophies,* by alopecia areata: *neoplastic,* by epithelioma: *hemorrhagic,* by purpura, ecchymoses, and bloody sweat: *infectious* diseases by erysipelas and syphilis, and even *microbic,* by furunculosis, abscess, and lupus.

It is not a little difficult to analyze the material presented accurately, and to determine or even suggest the exact manner in which the menstrual influence affects each or any of these; but it will be found that there is reasonable evidence that the result is produced in different manners in different diseases, and that each of the three conditions represented by the theories already alluded to, may be responsible for certain cases.

It must first be premised that in all this study of "the influence of the menstrual function on certain diseases of the skin" there is no claim whatever that such is the sole, efficient, operative *cause* in the production of skin lesions, except in rare instances, to be mentioned later. In many of the cases previously alluded to, the skin affection existed long previous to any observed changes which occurred during menstruation; and all of the eruptions may occur in males as well as in females, and most of them even in young children. But, as the cumulative clinical evidence is so very strong that certain changes in the skin may, and do often occur at or near the menstrual period, even in those with seemingly normal menstruation, the attempt is made to discover why this should happen. It is granted, of course, that the eruptions which are credited as appearing with or near menstruation, come only in those who are predisposed thereto, and, in part at least, from other causes, most of which are not definitely known. We may now consider the three theories and some of their relations to the diseases mentioned.

1. *Cyclic Changes in the General System.* In the opening chapter considerable attention was given to the "cyclic changes" noted by many observers as occurring in women and culminating at the menstrual epoch, which will now be further considered, with other matter.

All recognize and know that the menstruating woman, at least in the more highly civilized state and under the tension of modern life, is in many ways different from what she is at some portion or portions of the inter-menstrual period. A considerable number of women realize perfectly from their general feelings, or from some particular sensation, that the time of the flow is approaching, and would know of the occurrence of menstruation even without being aware of the actual flow having taken place; although a certain number often declare that they are quite unconscious of its occurrence. It may be safely said, however, that the majority of women, as met with in private practice in advanced civilization, experience sensations or conditions of the system, at or near the proper time of the menstrual flow, which are not experienced at other times. These are familiar to all, such as nervous irritability or incapacity for severe mental or muscular application; sensory disturbances, such as visual, aural, etc.; neuralgia, migraine, backache, aching of the limbs, and general abdominal sensations; as also fullness of the breasts, often with pain; while actual functional disturbances likewise often occur, such as constipation or intestinal and gastric disorders, as also those of the urinary tract. In addition to these there are many symptoms pertaining to the uterus and ovaries, varying from general abdominal uneasiness to agonizing cramps, great tenderness or pain in the ovaries, etc. Putnam-Jacobi[63] asserts, from the analysis of a large number of individuals that "in our existing social conditions, 46 per cent. of women suffer more or less during menstruation," referring to actual sexual discomfort. In view of all this, is it any wonder, therefore, that alterations should be observed in the skin in connection with the systemic changes resulting in menstruation?

In the opening chapter it was found that important changes take place in women in a rhythmical or cyclic manner. While there is a reduction of hæmoglobin and diminution of red cells, and slight increase of leucocytes, during the menstrual flow, it happens that in the inter-menstrual period the red cells slowly increase, reaching a maximum three days before the succeeding flow. The pulse is accelerated and the sphygmograph shows increased arterial tension during the seven to nine days preceding menstruation, and reaches a minimum point in from one to two days after its cessation.

There is an increase in weight up to the time of menstruation, and a sudden fall on its appearance; there is also a rise of temperature of about 1°F. during the increase in weight, in the week before menstruation, and a sudden fall of temperature after the crest of the wave has passed. The urea is generally increased in the urine before the appearance of the menses, and falls during and after; while the carbonic acid exhaled by the lungs is diminished during menstruation, and muscular strength is lessened. Changes also occur in the thyroid gland, and it is believed that there is a hypersecretion during menstruation.

These "cyclical changes," through which a woman passes each month, really in anticipation of pregnancy, culminate in the fatty degeneration of the hypertrophied uterine mucous membrane (no longer required for conception), and the consequent rupture of subjacent blood vessels, as Kundrat,[74] Williams,[124] Engelmann,[39] and others, have shown. For, as has been remarked, the menstrual flow is the least important part of the bodily process, which is recognized chiefly by this culminating feature of menstruation.

It is difficult to believe that all these changes in the system are caused by the ripening and discharge of the ovum, or that they depend in any manner upon the changes which go on in the uterus, ending in the menstrual discharge. It seems much more reasonable to agree with many observers that the "cyclic changes," which have been described, represent a development of surplus material and force each month, which is prepared for the ovum, if impregnated, and which is thrown off when not needed, by the menstrual discharge. Vrain[120] has called attention to the comparison of menstruation with pregnancy, which had been made previously by several writers, likening the menstrual discharge to a miniature confinement.

True it is that this monthly loss is but slight, from four to six ounces, but the ills resulting from a sudden checking of the flow, and also those from a failure of the system to undergo these changes, in amenorrhœa and chlorosis, give much support to the theory under consideration.

It would be quite beyond the scope of the present writing to consider the reason for this monthly explosion, which was formerly thought to be wholly due to the ripening and extrusion of the ovum. As it has been shown that ova are given off from early infancy, and also at other times than during menstruation, and even during prolonged amenorrhœa (Putnam-Jacobi), the true reason must still remain in doubt. Suffice it, however, to recognize that at periods of about a month apart, a climax is reached in the processes pertaining to female menstrual life, and that relief is given by a discharge from the reproductive organs, which, as Wagner[121] says, is "the elimination under a special form, of a superfluous productive material."

A good illustration of the necessity of relief to the systemic cyclical changes which take place occurred in my office very recently. Miss M., aged 53, a nervous and rather delicate lady, inclined to rheumatism, has had a number of severe illnesses, typhoid, etc., which kept her below par. About eight years ago she had ovariotomy performed, for a tumor, and has had no menses since that time, they having occurred regularly every 21 days previously. Since the operation, and the cessation of menses, she has had, every 21 days, symptoms of congestion, which invariably result in a sick headache, unless she makes free use of calomel, when they can be averted. This she has done, every three weeks, for some years.

An interesting confirmation of the tendency of the female to early cyclic changes is found in the many cases which have been reported of precocious menstruation, even from infancy.

Mannino[22] has recorded a curious and remarkable case which bears on this point. Liboria Bucalo, aged 10 years, had always been in good health, and had had no exanthematic fevers. Since the age of seven years she had had, each month. about the time of the full moon, an eruption on the right cheek. It began as a small lenticular spot of a bright red color, and gradually increased in area until at the end of eight or ten days it was about the size of a silver dollar; it then began to diminish and disappeared by the 13th or 14th day. For the first few years there was nothing to be seen in the intervals between the eruption, but after that the spot remained somewhat pigmented. The child was otherwise perfectly healthy: the heart was normal, there was no ovarian tenderness, and no leucorrhœa: she had never menstruated. Several photographs are given of the case, at different times.

Also the phenomena of vicarious menstruation, as shown by cases constantly reported by reliable observers, "of which Puech has collected two hundred, are proof positive of the existence in the female organism of a necessity for the periodical evacuation of a few ounces of blood" (Putnam Jacobi,[68] p. 103).

While we cannot, perhaps, speak of the conditions of system as indicated by the above, in the light of *causing* this or that disease of the skin, we can readily understand how, with an existing cutaneous disease such changes in metabolism and vascular tension should affect it more or less unfavorably; we can even conceive that with a predisposition to a certain skin lesion the conditions belonging to the "menstrual cycle" might act as an exciting cause of its appearance.

2. *Auto-intoxication of genital origin.* This explanation of the phenomena observed in various parts of the body, and applied especially to lesions of the skin by Goutry,[48] is interesting and more or less plausible.

Basing his arguments largely on the studies and observations of Charrin,[22] supported by others, he believes, First, that not only is there an auto-intoxication from failure of the menstruation to excrete certain poisons from the system, but also, Second, that the ovary is itself a secretory organ, and, in addition to providing the ovum, it acts in the same manner as the ductless organs, in furnishing some element to the blood, the absence of which can lead to auto-intoxication; as has been ably worked up by Howard Kelly.[70]

The first of these views has long been held, by many writers, the second, which has been ably supported by Spillman and Etienne;[106] Goutry[48] also argues strongly in favor of it as relating to skin lesions, from the action of ovarian and testicular extract in certain conditions, as reported by several observers. But in the absence of more definite knowledge it is hard to accept fully the theory that an ovarian secretion is the only or chief element which influences the system in the manner which has been already described. Our knowledge of the exact chemical and microscopical character of the menstrual fluid is also too slight to allow of the full acceptance of the theory of the imperfect elimination of toxic material thereby, as a cause of cutaneous and other disorders; although this works in very well with the previous theory of "cyclic changes" in the system, which require normal menstruation for their perfect completion.

Goutry very cleverly argues from the secretion of the kidney, which, while it may be normal in quantity and appearance, can yet be far from normal, and lead to intoxication. He also instances the toxicity of blood drawn from women about to menstruate, as shown by Charrin; likewise the well-known fact that the milk of women who begin to menstruate acts disadvantageously on the child, giving rise to intestinal disorders and even eruption on the skin.

3. *Nervous reflex irritation from the congested condition of the uterus and ovaries.* This third theory, as to the cause of the many symptoms accompanying menstruation, has much to commend it, as has been very fully shown by Engelmann,[39] whose observations I shall freely use. Although under the term "hystero-neuroses" he deals chiefly with the many disordered conditions of various parts of the

system which occur as a result of uterine or ovarian disease, he recognizes also the profound effect which menstruation may have in producing disorder or disease in distant organs, and devotes much attention to those on the skin.

In regard to menstrual hystero-neuroses he says: "I have so termed those neuroses which appear at the time of the menstrual congestion, but in few cases only are they determined by the physiological state pure and simple in a healthy organ. They are mostly dependent on changes, such as congestion or displacement, aggravated by the physiological conditions of menstruation, their peculiarity being that they come at this time only. They are often determined by pathological conditions, which in themselves are insufficient to bring about the neurosis, and only with the increased congestion or heightened nervous susceptibility accompanying the menstrual state does the neurosis appear. It is upon the congestion and the increased nervous excitability of the menstrual state that these neuroses depend, greater pressure, heightened functional activity, and greater susceptibility of the affected organ and its nerve fibres. Hence they appear, not at the time of the sanguineous flow, but during the entire period of congestion, beginning from two or three days to one week before the appearance of the flow, and passing away two or three days after its cessation, often disappearing during its continuance, while the depletion is in progress." He also considers largely the reflex neuroses occurring in connection with puberty, the menopause, and pregnancy, which need not detain us here.

But little is known in regard to the actual method in which affections of the skin may be influenced in a reflex manner by menstruation, or by uterine disease, but as there seems to be little question but that other organs may thus exhibit reflex action, it is reasonable to suppose that in certain instances neurotic influence may be thus exerted on the skin. The occurrence of actual skin lesions as a result of nerve influence is now well established, herpes zoster being a striking instance. In herpes gestationis[17] we have a conspicuous illustration of an active and intensely distressing eruption, of distinctly nervous character, recurring time and again with the gravid uterus and ceasing promptly when it is emptied: vesicular eczema is also known to recur on the hands as one of the early signs of pregnancy.

According to Engelmann, "the hystero-neurosis is a sympathetic hyperæsthesia, the result of reflex action due to uterine derangement: * * * it is a symptom which may be brought under the head of the gangliopathy of Tilt,[114] being determined by the various ramifications and connections of the ganglionic and spinal nerves and centers with the uterine and ovarian nerves. * * * Thus the irritation of the ganglionic nervous system caused by morbid changes in uterine and ovarian tissue, is most readily conveyed to the spinal and cerebral centers, following sometimes one, sometimes another path. * * * Most intimate is the connection of the ganglionic with the vaso-motor nerves: hence changes in the uterine tissue influence, through the ganglionic centers, the vaso-motor nerves, and produce either relaxation—which we often see made apparent by flushes, swelling, heat, and redness of the surface—or hyperactivity, marked by vascular contraction, by a chill or coldness of the extremities." While dwelling largely upon cutaneous disorders which depended upon uterine derangement, and which disappeared upon local uterine treatment, he often illustrates the effect of menstruation in causing the recurrence of the same.

In examining these three theories as to the manner in which menstruation may influence certain diseases of the skin, it is seen that they are not necessarily conflicting, indeed, that they are even complementary one to the other: and we shall see later that each may be properly invoked to explain some of the cutaneous phenomena observed in connection with menstruation, in certain cases.

But from what has preceded it would seem that the "cyclic changes" in the female organism which occur each month, as described, must be accepted as the bottom fact upon which to build any understanding of the cutaneous phenomena which have been recorded by so many observers in connection with menstruation.

This granted, it is easy to accept a part, at least, of the second theory, namely, auto-intoxication from faulty menstrual action; since some of the skin disorders, as Behrend[6] suggests, bear such a striking resemblance to eruptions caused by infectious processes or by drugs. Whether the ovary is a secretory organ (other than for ova), and whether its faulty secretion induces trouble in other organs, as described by some, in the second theory, is as yet somewhat problematical, and need hardly be wholly accepted, inasmuch as the phenomena supposed to be thus produced are explainable on other grounds.

The third theory, that of *reflex nervous irritation* from the reproductive organs, follows very naturally from what has preceded. All are acquainted with the various reflex symptoms, often so puzzling, which result from uterine and ovarian diseases, and there can be little doubt but that all portions of the system may be thus affected. We have seen that material changes are continually going on in the uterine mu-

cous membrane, and we know that the uterus and
ovary are in a state of turgidity and nervous excita-
tion before and during menstruation, which are easily
explained, both as a result of the general vascular
tension belonging to the "cyclic changes" described,
and also from their own physiological activity at this
period. In the monthly elimination from the uterus
of the surplus material, which is quite possibly of
a toxic character, it is very natural that nervous excitement should occur, which by natural laws can
readily be reflected elsewhere.

Applying these principles to the various cutaneous
conditions which have been mentioned as influenced
by menstruation, we can see that effects may be produced in each of the three methods specified.

Foremost must stand the "cyclic changes" under-
gone by the system, whereby a surplus of nutritive,
and possibly imperfectly elaborated material is cir-
culating in the blood, with high arterial tension,
slight rise of temperature, etc. The congestive and
inflammatory dermatoses, such as eczema and others,
would readily take on exaggerated action under these
conditions, and with a strong disposition to them
they could easily be excited to active or renewed development: the same applies to an inflammatory
glandular disease such as acne. It is also quite un-
derstandable that such a condition of blood as de-

scribed, where "the red cells slowly increase, reaching a maximum three days before the menstrual flow," would also be effective in modifying many of the other diseases of the skin which have been recorded as influenced by menstruation.

It is not difficult to understand even how microbic diseases may be influenced by the process of the system which ends in what is known as menstruation. It is well recognized that the micro-cocci which belong to suppuration are almost omnipresent, and yet how few, comparatively, suffer from boils, carbuncles, and abscesses. As in the case of the bacilli of tuberculosis, it is well known that all micro-organisms flourish only on a suitable soil, and cannot be cultivated except in proper media and under suitable conditions; also that certain individuals seem peculiarly exempt from their invasion, however much exposed, just as many escape infectious diseases. It is only necessary to recognize that, under certain conditions, the peculiar state of system represented by these "cyclic changes" affords the proper nidus for the micro-organism to flourish in and the matter is clear, even in regard to erysipelas. Possibly also the lowered state of vitality, belonging to this period, as shown by the advent of many diseases, may render the system and the tissues less able to resist the attack of micro-organisms, and the leucocytes less equal to the task of defending the body against them.

It is undoubtedly true that many of the cases which are often regarded as erysipelas of menstruation are quite other conditions, rosaceous acne, erythema, erythematous eczema, and pseudo-erysipelas, excited or developed under the influence of the menstrual state. But there have been many cases recorded, as already mentioned, where true, febrile erysipelas of infectious character has been observed to recur with each menstruation, and recent writers on menstrual erysipelas, Tourneux,[116] Cachera,[19] and Salvy,[102] recognize fully the streptococcic origin of erysipelas, so that there is no question but that many of the cases observed were of this nature.

The relations of infection to menstruation in these cases can be better understood in the light of some recent observations of Petit.[98] He reports twelve cases of streptococcal sore throat occurring at the menstrual epoch, sometimes repeatedly in the same woman. Virulent streptoccocci, capable of causing erysipelas when inoculated into rabbits' ears, were found in the secretions of the throat in each case. The time of appearance of the sore throat varied, sometimes coinciding with the menstrual period, sometimes preceding it by a few days. The author believed that the streptococci were in the throat, in a quiescent condition, but became active when the disturbances associated with menstruation rendered the soil suitable. "We know well to-day," says he, "that the menstrual epoch brings about modifications in the circulation of the mucous membranes. * * * Furthermore, every one recognizes the fact that the woman is in a condition of functional inferiority during menstruation; she is at that time more susceptible to the attacks of infectious agents and is also less able to defend herself against them."

Goutry[48] quotes Genet[44] in regard to a tonsillitis periodically accompanying normal and regular menstruation. In certain cases, under the influence of a sudden arrest of the menses, the symptoms are more acute and sometimes terminate in suppuration. He also mentions Gautier[48] as having examined bacteriologically and finding streptococci, in six cases of menstrual angina, which he studied.

Many writers have believed that an element in the ultimate causation of all cases of erysipelas is found in certain conditions of the nervous and circulatory system (Roger[99]) which have been observed to exert an influence on the development of the streptococcus. As these disturbances belong to the menstrual state it is readily seen that the third, or reflex nervous hypothesis, may aid in explaining the recurrence of erysipelas at the menstrual period: for it is recognized that the streptococcus, while not omnipresent as some other cocci, is not an infrequent habitant of even healthy persons.

The third or *nervous reflex* hypothesis of the influence of menstruation finds much confirmation in connection with certain troubles of the skin. Thus the abundant flushings and perspiration observed at the menopause, and not infrequently with menstruation, are evidently of neurotic origin, and it is easy to understand how uterine and ovarian irritation can cause such, by reflex operation through the vasomotor nerves. All recognize that ordinary blushing is of nervous character, and the perspiration which can start so freely on fright or excitement is known to all.

It is more than likely that the herpes, which we have seen to develop so frequently with menstruation, is wholly neurotic, as also the pemphigus, which has been described. The same is probably true in regard to purpura, ecchymoses, and bloody sweat. The pruritus accompanying menstruation may be wholly reflex or due to the gradual increase of vascular tension during the inter-menstrual period; and its maximum just before the menstrual flow, may be the result of the "cyclic changes," as we know that the itching of many eruptions is increased by heightened vascular activity.

The second theory, that of auto-intoxication of genital origin, may also explain some of the phenomena observed in the skin. Although, as previously remarked, this matter is still somewhat problematical, it is worthy of our consideration. Keiffer[68] has argued strongly in favor of it, and others have also maintained the same. He says: "Menstruation is not a local function, but is a means of elimination of certain internal secretions—it is not a hemorrhage, or a simple sanguineous extravasation, but it is a true excretion; suppression of menstruation induces symptoms analogous to those resulting from suppression of the renal secretion—there is a menorrhæmia comparable to uræmia. The symptoms arising from suppression of menstruation are chiefly of two kinds—vaso-motor and nervous. In the first group we have passive congestion of the pelvic organs and of the entire intestine: palpitations, hot flushes, muscæ volitantes, sudden pallor and flushing, cold sweats, exaggerated secretion of the cutaneous glands, congestion of cicatrices, and lesions of the skin. In the second group are, anorexia, nausea, vomiting, headache, depression, painful zones in various parts of the body, etc." Others speak of retained secretions which defective menstruation has failed to eliminate.

The chloasma of pregnancy has been ascribed by

certain writers to changes in the coloring matter of the blood, due to some poison not eliminated by the arrested menstruation, and it is possible that some of the pigmentary conditions seen with menstruation (which may be defective) are from this cause. If there be such a thing as auto-intoxication of genital origin it is quite possible that it may enter to a greater or less extent into the influences of menstruation in many of the cutaneous affections mentioned.

We have thus endeavored to account for some of the conditions of the skin which have been observed during menstruation, but recognize that much work, experimental and clinical, must yet be done before the subject is as clear as could be desired.

One thing is certain, and that is, that abundant evidence has been collected and recorded to show that certain diseases of the skin are often influenced in a striking manner in connection with menstruation. It is clear that these changes take place in the ten days just before and including the menstrual flow, and that they often appear with very great regularity. That they do not always thus happen is no argument against the true relationship, for it is quite possible that when they fail to occur the menstrual flow has been more nearly that of perfect functioning; this latter occurrence may point strongly to the second theory, of auto-intoxication, when they do occur. We certainly need far more observation and study in regard to the exact character of the menstrual flow under various conditions.

CHAPTER IV.

TREATMENT.

To accept what some have written one might think that all the external phenomena occurring in connection with menstruation were to be relieved only by proper, local gynæcological treatment. But from long and very considerable experience with the conditions occurring on the skin, as already detailed, I feel very certain that this is not the case. On the other hand, I believe that it is often useless, or unnecessary, in most cases where menstrual influences in diseases of the skin are apparent, to attempt local treatment to the sexual organs alone, without due regard to other matters, to be mentioned later: for in dozens of instances I have known this to have previously failed lamentably in patients who have subsequently come under my care.

Undoubtedly when there is marked uterine or ovarian disease they are to be recognized and properly treated, and in a certain number of instances this will have a markedly beneficial effect upon the eruption. But in a large share of the cases, at least of those which have come under my observation, the disorders of menstruation which have seemed to have some influence in causing or aggravating skin lesions are mainly those of the functional class, and the amenorrhœa, dysmenorrhœa, menorrhagia, and leucorrhœa have been largely symptoms of an anæmia or abdominal congestion, commonly resulting from disorders of the digestive and urinary organs.

It is also to be remembered that as a rule the menstrual element is only one single factor in regard to the eruption. There are often many points to be considered, and treatment can be successful only as it is based on the broadest lines of medical knowledge and judgment. While the menstrual element may sometimes seem to be very important it need generally be no bar to the successful treatment of the eruption: for under a careful and intelligent treatment of the general condition, and of the eruption, by dietetic, hygienic, and medicinal means, both the skin disorder and any associated menstrual derangement will often cease. For the menstrual influence on the eruption is only the result of some derangement farther back in the life processes of the body, which must be reached if any treatment is to be effectual.

It is readily seen, therefore, that local treatment to the skin must also play a relatively unimportant part in the management of many of these cases. While this may give much relief, and often render signal aid in overcoming the local difficulty, its effects can be but local, and as long as the underlying cause remains its benefits will be but temporary. The local treatment of these eruptions does not differ from that proper to similar lesions of ordinary type, and need not detain us here.

The internal treatment naturally differs greatly with the disease and with the particular case, and cannot be specified in full. But there are certain underlying principles which can be dwelt on with advantage.

As already intimated, the menstrual influence is exhibited in certain diseases of the skin because there are faults in the life processes of the economy which are intensified by the "cyclic changes" which culminate at menstruation, and by the nervous irritability produced by the congested reproductive organs. These errors of function belong to a number of different organs, or to an associated disturbance of several of them.

First to be mentioned is imperfect action of the bowels. This is such a trite subject that it is difficult to write upon it clearly and effectually in a few words, but its importance is so great in this connection that it must receive considerable attention.

With many the habit of constipation is so common that it seems quite a natural thing, and previous efforts at its removal have often been so ineffective that it is only by the utmost care that proper attention to it can be secured. But from long observation I am convinced that with great diligence and patience on the part of the physician and patient the desired result, of a thoroughly proper, daily, morning evacuation of the bowels, can be secured. It is not enough simply to inquire at the beginning of treatment if the bowels are regular, but frequent inquiry must be made and proper means be employed to obtain the desired result.

It is not enough to give purgative or laxative remedies occasionally, nor to leave the matter to the discretion of the individual, but each step must be directed with patient care until the desired end is attained. I am not in favor of enemata or suppositories for this purpose, nor of the mineral waters, or the phosphate of soda, neither do I care for the salts so commonly used, but believe that the proper use of vegetable laxatives conforms more to the processes of nature.

But there are often other disturbances of the intestinal tract which require to be looked into and rectified; for intestinal indigestion is often at the bottom of many skin affections, and may produce disturbance of the reproductive organs. And this should also not be lightly regarded, but carefully investigated and treated intelligently and persistently.

As is well known, many of these disturbances are due to gastric disorders, and these, in turn, to faulty diet and mode of life, whereby also liver derangement adds to the accumulated errors. This is not the place to enter fully into the consideration of these matters, but they are often of such vital importance that they should constantly receive the most searching and careful investigation and consideration. In all these matters, as indeed in much pertaining to medical practice, it is well to go on the presumption that the patient knows little or nothing accurately, and to hold such a control over everything pertaining to health that the desired end shall surely be accomplished.

Disturbances of the kidney function are not at all uncommon in connection with the class of cases which have been considered, and are often to be regarded only as an indication of the manner in which the processes of metabolism are carried on. It is not common to find albumen or sugar in the urine of these patients, but there are frequently very gross variations from health in regard to the specific gravity, acidity, urea, indican, and the various salts found normally, while uric acid, urates, oxalate of lime and phosphates are often present, microscopically. All of these have their significance, which should certainly be considered and acted upon in order to obtain satisfactory results. The urinary and reproductive organs are very closely related, biologically, anatomically, physiologically, and pathologically, as Etheridge[39] has so excellently shown, saying, "Very many gynæcological patients suffer greatly from renal insufficiency, and properly selected diuretics will relieve many of their symptoms commonly referred to the reflexes from pelvic maladies." This again is a subject worthy of elaboration, in this connection, but cannot be entered on fully.

In many patients exhibiting a menstrual influence in certain diseases of the skin, it will be found that anæmia is really the principal factor in all the troubles, even those relating to the sexual organs. But again, quite as frequently, careful study will show that this anæmia is only the result of some of the conditions which have been already specified. In such cases it is often worse than useless to give iron alone, but when the functions of digestion and excretion have been properly attended to, it will prove most effective.

In approaching a case exhibiting menstrual influences in any disease of the skin we must, therefore, take a very broad view of the subject. It will not answer simply to prescribe local treatment for the skin lesion present, nor, on the other hand to treat only any real or supposed sexual disorder locally, with a view of remedying the cutaneous ailment. Careful study demonstrates that there are many causes which must be searched out and rectified, in order to obtain satisfactory results. Each case must be carefully studied on its own merits, and suitable treatment, dietary, hygienic and medicinal, applied, with, of course, proper gynæcological measures when they are plainly indicated.

BIBLIOGRAPHY.

1. Alibert, Précis théoret. et prat., Paris, 1818, Vol. I, p. 410.
2. Anderson, McCall, Jour. of Cutaneous Med., Vol. I, 1878, p. 328.
3. Banks, Dublin Quar. Jour. of Med. Science, 1858, p. 257.
4. Batuand, Rev. Medico-Chir. des mal. des femmes, 1886, VIII, p. 260.
5. Behrend, Lehrb. der Hautkrankheiten, Berlin, 1883, pp. 188, 314.
6. Belfield, Jour. Amer. Med. Assn., June 13, 1903, p. 1653.
7. Bergh, Herpes menstrualis, Monatsh. für prat. Dermat., 1890, p. 13.
8. Billard, Archives gén. de Méd., 1831, p. 453.
9. Bloom, Arch. Pediatrics, New York, 1897, XIV, p. 693.
10. Bohn, Deut. med Arch. für klin. med., October, 1886.
11. Bouchard, Leçons sur la thérap. des mal. infect., Paris, 1889, p. 286.
12. Börner, Volkmann's Sammlung, 1886, No. 312.
13. Brocq, Ann. de Derm. et de Syph., 1888, p. 210.
14. Bruneau, Thèse de Paris, 1880, p. 42.
15. Bulkley, Acne, its Etiology, Pathology and Treatment, New York, 1885, p. 71.
16. Bulkley, Eczema, 3d Edit., Putnam, New York, 1901, p. 10.
17. Bulkley, Am. Journ. Obstet. and Diseases of Women and Children, Vol. VI, 1874.
18. Byers, Lancet, 1899, II, p. 553.
19. Cachera, De l'érysipèle a répétition, Thèse de Paris, 1891.
20. Cazal, Dictionnaire Encyclop. des Sci. Med.
21. Chausit, Ann. des Mal. de la Peau, Vol. IV, 1851, p. 118.
22. Charrin, La chlorose. Gaz. hebdom. 2 Jan., 1896; also, Leçon de pathogénie appliquée, p. 178, quoted by Goutry, pp. 60 et seq.

23. Clairborne, Jour. Amer. Med. Assn., 1902, p. 631.
24. Coughlin, Med. Record, Vol. LIII, 1898, p. 805.
25. Cummings, British Med. Jour., 1884, Part II, p. 20.
26. Currier, New York Journal of Gynæcol., 1892, p. 55; 1893, p. 48.
27. Danlos, Étude sur la menstruation, au point de vue de son influence sur les mal. cutan., Paris, 1874.
28. DeKeyser, Ann. de Derm. et de Syph., 1903, p. 704.
29. Deligny, Jour. Cut. and Gen.-ur. Dis., 1888, p. 319.
30. Deligny, La Concourse Médicale, April 14, 1888.
31. Diday and Doyon, Les herpes génitaux, Paris, 1886, pp. 128, 296.
32. Dolgonoff, Vratch, St. Petersburg, 1900, XXI, p. 1107.
33. Dubreuilh, Annales de Derm. et de Syph., 1903, p. 167.
34. Duhring and Hartzell, Keating's Clin. Gynæc., Philadelphia, 1895, p. 980.
35. Duhring, The Medical News, Philadelphia, July 19, 1884.
36. Du Mesnil de Rochemont, Arch. für Derm. & Syph., XXX, 1895, p. 190.
37. Duncan, The Lancet, London, 1881, I, p. 53.
38. Edebohls, N. Y. Jour. of Gyn. and Obstet., 1892, p. 55, 1893, p. 48.
39. Engelmann, G. J., The hystero-neuroses, Gyn. Trans., New York, 1887.
40. Etheridge, Trans. Med. Soc. of the State of N. Y., 1896, p. 104.
41. Ewing, Clinical pathology of the blood, Philadelphia, 1901, p. 90.
42. Fox, Long, The Influence of the Sympathetic on Disease, London, 1885.
43. Gautier, Des angines de la menstruation, Thèse de Paris, 1894—5.
44. Genet, Consid. Clin. et phys. * * * des amygdales pendant menstr., Paris, 1881. (Quoted by Goutry.)
45. Gerson, Ann. de Dermat. et de Syph., 1897, p. 1180.
46. Gillet, Annales de la Policlinique de Paris, II, 1892, p. 320.
47. Godot, De l'érysipèle menstruel, Thèse de Paris, 1883.
48. Goutry, De l'infl. de la menstr. sur les affect. cut., Thèse de Paris, 1899 (good bibliography).
49. Grecken, Frauenarzt, Berlin, 1887, II, p. 195.

50. Green, American Journal of Otology, April, 1881.
51. Greenough, Arch. of Dermatology, Vol. VII, 1881, pp. 14, 69, 70.
52. Grelletty, De l'érysipèle lié a la menstruation, Gaz. Obstet., 1878, p. 113.
53. Grelletty, Wood's Med. and Surg. Monographs, New York, 1889.
54. Guibout, Traité prat. des mal. de la Peau, Paris, 1885, p. 273.
55. Hardy, Leçons sur les Mal. de la Peau, Paris, 1863, p. 32.
56. Hardy, Traité prat. et descr. des Mal. de la Peau, Paris, 1886, p. 269.
57. Hebra, Lehrb. der Hautkr., 2d Edit., Erlangen, 1874, Vol. I, pp. 457, 462, 631.
58. Hebra, Wochenbl. der Zeitsch. der Gesell. d. Aerzte, No. 40, 1855.
59. Hebra, Lehrb. der Hautkr., Erlangen, 2d Edit., 1874, Vol. I, p. 262b.
60. Hebra, Quoted in Keating and Coe, Clinical Gynæc., Philadelphia, 1895, p. 984.
61. Hirst, Barton, Gynæcology, New York, 1895, p. 83.
62. Hobbs, Arch. clin. de Bordeaux, 1892, p. 38.
63. Jacobi, Putnam, Rest during menstruation, New York, 1886, p. 143 et seq.
64. Jamieson, Diseases of the Skin, 3d Edit., Philadelphia, 1892, p. 454.
65. Janowsky and Schwing, Centrabl. für Gynæk., 1882, VI, No. 17, p. 257.
66. Joseph, Berliner klin. Wochensch. No. 37, 1879, p. 554.
67. Keating and Coe, Clinical Gynæcology, Philadelphia, 1895, p. 772.
68. Keiffer, L'Obstetrique, Paris, July 15, 1897.
69. Keiffer, La Presse Médicale Belge, 1897, pp. 249, 257.
70. Kelly, Howard, Operative Gynæcology, New York, 1899, Vol. II, p. 165.
71. Kelsey, Med. Record, 1892, Vol. XLI, p. 77.
72. Kerr, Virginia Medical Monthly, Vol. 13, 1886-7, p. 704.
73. Kidd, Proceed. Dublin Obstet. Soc. (Cited by Engelmann, p. 129.)
74. Kundrat, Stricker's Med. Jahrb., 1873, Heft. 2, quoted by Putnam Jacobi, p. 92.

75. Laredde, Ann. de Dermat. et de Syph., 1899, p. 130.
76. Laussedat, Ann. de Derm. et de Syph., 1891, p. 407.
77. Legendre, Arch. Gén. de Méd., 1853, Vol. II, p. 171.
78. Leveque, Dermatoses d'origine nerveuse, etc., Thèse de Lillie, 1887, p. 36.
79. Leroy de Mericourt, Archives gén. de Méd., 1857, p. 430.
80. Liégeois, Revue méd. de l'est, Vol. XI, p. 460.
81. Loewenberg, Progrès médicale, 1881, p. 633.
82. McGillicuddy, Functional disorders of the nervous system in women, New York, 1898, p. 77.
83. Mannino, Atti della R. Accad. della Scienze Mediche Palermo, 1898.
84. Massalongo, La Riforma Medica, 1894, IV, p. 39.
85. Mitchell, Weir, Fat and Blood, Lippincott, Philadelphia, 1877, p. 13.
86. Morin, Purpura simpl. catamenial, Bulletin Med., 1891. (Quoted by Goutry, p. 47.)
87. Moses, Amer. Jour. Med. Sci., Vol. 38, 1859, p. 357.
88. Moutard-Martin, Des accid. qui accomp. l'établ. de la mens. Thèse de Paris, 1846, p. 15.
89. Neligan, Dublin Quar. Jour. de Med. Sci., 1855, p. 293.
90. Nicolaysen, J., Festskr. Prof. Herberg's, Kristiania, 1895, p. 196.
91. Parvin, Gynæcological Transactions, Vol. I, p. 135.
92. Pauli, Berliner klin. Wochenschr., 1880, XVII, p. 646.
93. Petit, Raymond, Streptococque et menstruation. Gaz. heb. de méd. et de chir., 1895, pp. 55 & 66.
94. Polotebnoff, Monatsch. f. prakt. Dermat., 1887, Erganz. Hefte II.
95. Putnam-Jacobi, see Jacobi.
96. Quincke, Monatsch. f. prakt. Dermat., Bd. I, 1882, p. 129.
97. Rayer, Traité théor. et prat. des Mal. de la Peau, Paris, 1835, Vol. I, pp. 147, 273, 400.
98. Roger, Comptes rendus Soc. Biologie, 1891-92.
99. Roger, Quoted by Salvy, q.v., p. 39.
100. Rohé, Buffalo Med. and Surg. Journal, February, 1889.
101. Royer, Collard, Thèse de 26 Thermidor, Ann. X. (Quoted by Goutry, p. 44.)
102. Salvy, Les Rapports de la Menstruation et de l'érysipèle, Paris, 1896.

103. Sanctorius, Aphorism LXV, 1770. (Quoted by Putnam-Jacobi, l. c., p. 9.)
104. Scanzoni, Quoted by Hanfield Jones, Functional Nerv. Disorders, 1864, p. 463.
105. Schramm, Berliner klin. Wochenschr., 1878, XV, p. 626.
106. Spillman and Etienne, Rev. med de l'Est, 1896, No. 21. (Quoted by Goutry, p. 66.)
107. Stiller, Berliner klin. Wochenschr., 1877, XIV, p. 731.
108. Süsemihl, Deutsche Klinik, Berlin, 1851, III, p. 87.
109. Tait, Quoted by Rohé, Buff. Med. and Surg. Jour., Feb., 1889.
110. Tedrowe, Med. Councillor, 1902, VII, p. 406.
111. Teevan, Medico-Chir. Trans. of London, 1845, Vol. 28.
112. Thirial, Jour. de Méd. de Trousseau, 1845.
113. Thomas, De l'érysipèle periodique catamenial, Paris, 1878.
114. Tilt, The Change of Life, 4th Edit., Philadelphia, 1882, pp. 83-102.
115. Tommasoli, Jour. des mal. cutan. et Syph., Vol. VII, 1895, p. 449; also, Gior. ital. delle mal. ven. e della pelle, 1895, pp. 33, 160.
116. Tourneux, De l'érysipèle catamenial, Thèse de Paris, 1886.
117. Townsend, Boston Med. and Surg. Jour., 1800, CXXIII, p. 516.
118. Tyrrell, Medical Record, 1897, Vol. LII. p. 160.
119. Unna, Journ. of Cutan. and Ven. Dis., New York, 1883, pp. 322, 328.
120. Vrain, La Menstruation * * * avec quelq. manif. cutanées, Thèse de Paris, 1878.
121. Wagner, Allgem. med. Centralzeit., Berlin, XLVII, p. 1173.
122. Wagner, Handworterbuch, Bd. IV, p. 879, 1853. (Quoted by Putnam Jacobi, p. 11.)
123. Wilhelm, Berliner klin. Wochenschr., 1878, XIV, p. 50.
124. Williams, London Obstet. Jour. (Quoted by Putnam Jacobi, pp. 92, 94.)
125. Wilson, Erasmus. Jour. Cutan. Med., Vol. III, 1869, p. 308.
126. Yonge, Philosoph. Transact., 1709.

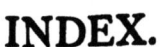

INDEX.

INDEX.

CPSIA information can be obtained
at www.ICGtesting.com
Printed in the USA
BVHW04s1029210918
528173BV00023B/1586/P